THE TEACHING OF DYNAMIC PSYCHIATRY

A Reappraisal of the Goals and Techniques in the Teaching of Psychoanalytic Psychiatry

Proceedings of the Symposium
held in Cambridge, Massachusetts
October 30 and 31, 1964

Sponsored by the
Psychiatric Service
Grete L. Bibring, Chief of Service
Beth Israel Hospital
Boston, Massachusetts

THE TEACHING OF DYNAMIC PSYCHIATRY

A Reappraisal of the Goals and Techniques in the Teaching of Psychoanalytic Psychiatry

edited by
GRETE L. BIBRING, M.D.

Symposium Committee

HENRY G. ALTMAN, M.D., *Chairman*
RALPH J. KAHANA, M.D.
ARTHUR R. KRAVITZ, M.D.
CAVIN P. LEEMAN, M.D.
JOHN VORENBERG, M.D.
NORMAN E. ZINBERG, M.D.

HARRIET H. GIBNEY, *Editorial Assistant*

Contributors

BERNARD BANDLER, M.D., Professor of Psychiatry, Chairman, Division of Psychiatry, Boston University School of Medicine

GRETE L. BIBRING, M.D., Psychiatrist-in-Chief, Beth Israel Hospital, and Clinical Professor of Psychiatry, Faculty of Medicine, Harvard University

DOUGLAS D. BOND, M.D., Professor of Psychiatry and Dean, School of Medicine, Western Reserve University

THOMAS F. DWYER, M.D., Associate Director, Psychiatric Service, Beth Israel Hospital, and Assistant Clinical Professor of Psychiatry, Faculty of Medicine, Harvard University

[v]

CONTRIBUTORS

ERIK H. ERIKSON, Professor of Human Development, Harvard University, and Instructor in Psychiatry, Faculty of Medicine, Harvard University

JACK R. EWALT, M.D., Superintendent, Massachusetts Mental Health Center, and Bullard Professor of Psychiatry, Faculty of Medicine, Harvard University

HENRY M. FOX, M.D., Physician, Peter Bent Brigham Hospital, and Associate Clinical Professor of Psychiatry, Faculty of Medicine, Harvard University

GEORGE E. GARDNER, M.D., Director, Judge Baker Guidance Center, and Psychiatrist-in-Chief, The Children's Hospital Medical Center, and Clinical Professor of Psychiatry, Faculty of Medicine, Harvard University

MAXWELL GITELSON, M.D.,* Chicago, Illinois; President, International Psychoanalytic Association, and Past President, American Psychoanalytic Association

THEODORE JACOBS, M.D., Instructor in Psychiatry, Albert Einstein College of Medicine

RALPH J. KAHANA, M.D., Associate Visiting Psychiatrist, Beth Israel Hospital, and Clinical Associate in Psychiatry, Faculty of Medicine, Harvard University

M. RALPH KAUFMAN, M.D., Director, Department of Psychiatry, The Mount Sinai Hospital, New York; Clinical Professor of Psychiatry, Columbia University College of Physicians and Surgeons, and Past President, American Psychoanalytic Association

LAWRENCE S. KUBIE, M.D., Clinical Professor of Psychiatry, University of Maryland, and Lecturer in Psychiatry, Johns Hopkins University

* Deceased

Erich Lindemann, M.D., Psychiatrist-in-Chief, Massachusetts General Hospital, and Professor of Psychiatry, Faculty of Medicine, Harvard University

Rudolph M. Loewenstein, M.D., New York City; Past President, American Psychoanalytic Association

Joseph J. Michaels, M.D.,* Visiting Psychiatrist, Beth Israel Hospital, and Past President, Boston Psychoanalytic Society and Institute

Paul G. Myerson, M.D., Psychiatrist-in-Chief, Tufts New England Medical Center, and Professor and Chairman, Department of Psychiatry, Tufts University School of Medicine

Sanford Oxenhorn, M.D., Instructor in Psychiatry and Medicine, Albert Einstein College of Medicine

Gregory Rochlin, M.D., Director and Chief of Service, Child Psychiatry, Massachusetts Mental Health Center, and Associate Clinical Professor of Psychiatry, Faculty of Medicine, Harvard University

Milton Rosenbaum, M.D., Professor and Chairman, Department of Psychiatry, Albert Einstein College of Medicine

Albert J. Solnit, M.D., Psychiatrist-in-Chief, Yale University Child Study Center

Alfred H. Stanton, M.D., Psychiatrist-in-Chief, The McLean Hospital, and Associate Professor of Psychiatry, Faculty of Medicine, Harvard University

Malvina Stock, M.D., Associate Visiting Psychiatrist, Beth Israel Hospital, and Training Analyst, Boston Psychoanalytic Society and Institute

Helen H. Tartakoff, M.D., Associate Visiting Psychiatrist, Beth Israel Hospital; Training Analyst, Boston Psychoanalytic Society and Institute

* Deceased

CHARLES W. TIDD, M.D., Professor of Psychiatry and Head, Division of Adult Psychiatry, University of California School of Medicine, Los Angeles

ARTHUR F. VALENSTEIN, M.D., Associate Visiting Psychiatrist, Beth Israel Hospital, and Training Analyst, Boston Psychoanalytic Society and Institute

HENRY WERMER, M.D., Head, Child Psychiatric Unit, Beth Israel Hospital, and Clinical Associate in Psychiatry, Faculty of Medicine, Harvard University

ELIZABETH R. ZETZEL, M.D., Psychiatrist, Massachusetts General Hospital, The McLean Hospital, and Assistant Clinical Professor of Psychiatry, Faculty of Medicine, Harvard University

NORMAN E. ZINBERG, M.D., Assistant Director, Psychiatric Service, Beth Israel Hospital; Assistant Clinical Professor of Psychiatry, Faculty of Medicine, Harvard University

Guests

HELENE DEUTSCH, M.D., Training Analyst Emeritus, Boston Psychoanalytic Society and Institute, and Honorary Professor of Psychology, Boston University

FRANK HAENDEL, M.D., Resident, Massachusetts General Hospital—The McLean Hospital

SILVIO J. ONESTI, JR., M.D., Head of Child Psychiatry Unit, Beth Israel Hospital, and Instructor in Psychiatry, Harvard Medical School

JOHN P. SPIEGEL, M.D., Associate Clinical Professor of Psychiatry, Faculty of Medicine, Harvard University, and Lecturer, Department of Social Relations, Harvard University

Contents

GRETE L. BIBRING—*Preface* 1

GRETE L. BIBRING—*Can Psychiatry Be Taught?* 5

Panel I. Medical Students
Chairman: GRETE L. BIBRING

THOMAS F. DWYER—*Psychoanalytic Teaching in the Medical School* 23

CHARLES W. TIDD—*Teaching Dynamic Psychiatry to Medical Students* 38

Invited Discussion

  BERNARD BANDLER 56

  DOUGLAS D. BOND 62

  ALFRED H. STANTON 68

General Discussion: LAWRENCE S. KUBIE, MILTON ROSENBAUM, ALBERT J. SOLNIT, CHARLES W. TIDD, THOMAS F. DWYER, FRANK HAENDEL, THEODORE JACOBS, ARTHUR F. VALENSTEIN, GREGORY ROCHLIN 71

Panel II. Psychiatric Residents
Chairman: HELEN H. TARTAKOFF

RALPH J. KAHANA—*Psychotherapy: Models of the Essential Skill* 87

RUDOLPH M. LOEWENSTEIN—*Psychoanalytic Theory and the Teaching of Dynamic Psychiatry* 104

Invited Discussion

  MAXWELL GITELSON 116

  LAWRENCE S. KUBIE 118

  GREGORY ROCHLIN 122

  ELIZABETH R. ZETZEL 126

[ix]

CONTENTS

General Discussion: DOUGLAS D. BOND, ARTHUR F. VALENSTEIN, RALPH J. KAHANA, RUDOLPH M. LOEWEN-STEIN 131

Panel III. Physicians in the Community
Chairman: JOSEPH J. MICHAELS

HENRY WERMER AND MALVINA STOCK—*"I Am Just a Pediatrician": Educating Pediatricians in Dynamic Psychiatry* 143

ALBERT J. SOLNIT—*Eight Pediatricians and a Child Psychiatrist: A Study in Collaboration* 158

Invited Discussion
    JACK R. EWALT 175
    GEORGE E. GARDNER 180
    M. RALPH KAUFMAN 185
    ERICH LINDEMANN 188

General Discussion: JOHN P. SPIEGEL, SILVIO J. ONESTI, JR., HENRY WERMER 190

Panel IV. House Officers
Chairman: ARTHUR F. VALENSTEIN

NORMAN E. ZINBERG—*The Problem of Values in Teaching Psychoanalytic Psychiatry* 203

MILTON ROSENBAUM, with THEODORE JACOBS and SANFORD OXENHORN—*Medical Students, Medical Residents, and Family Physicians* 226

Invited Discussion
    ERIK H. ERIKSON 247
    HENRY M. FOX 252
    PAUL G. MYERSON 257

General Discussion: MILTON ROSENBAUM, ALBERT J. SOLNIT, JOHN P. SPIEGEL, HELENE DEUTSCH 263

Bibliography 271

Preface

THE PLAN FOR THIS SYMPOSIUM has grown out of 20 years of activities on the psychiatric service at the Beth Israel Hospital in Boston. It represents an attempt to review the different trends in an area of our special interest—teaching psychiatry to physicians, medical students, and psychiatric residents.

After World War II, physicians and psychiatrists returned to civilian life with an increased awareness of the psychological complications of organic illnesses and the psychogenesis of certain conditions which seemed to be of an organic nature. Hermann Blumgart, Physician-in-Chief of the Beth Israel Hospital, was one of those who gave determined support to the development of a strong department of psychiatry which, in addition to its own program, would teach psychiatric principles to doctors and medical students in a general hospital. As the newly appointed head of this department, I was fortunate in having the active cooperation of my late husband, Dr. Edward Bibring, and of a small group of colleagues, many of whom were close friends and associates. Doctors Martin Berezin, Leo Berman, Louis Chase, Joseph J. Michaels,

[1]

Paul G. Myerson, and Helen H. Tartakoff were members of the staff in 1946.

From 1946 to 1950 this group devoted itself to the novel and interesting assignment of teaching psychiatry within a general hospital. We were joined by Doctors Lydia Dawes, Thomas F. Dwyer, Sidney Levin, Cecil Mushatt, Arthur F. Valenstein, Henry Wermer, and Norman E. Zinberg. We had a common bond of interest and experience, and we had all been trained in psychoanalysis. The challenges we faced were twofold. First, we had to learn to apply what we had learned from individual psychoanalytic therapy to medicine and the different areas of specialized medicine; then we had to find ways to teach this in a usable and constructive form to physicians, medical students, social workers, and nurses. The continuing devoted and competent contributions of these psychiatrists make our service what it is today.

As of 1950 the department has grown steadily. In 1955 it became an independent fifth service of the Hospital, in addition to medicine, surgery, pediatrics, and obstetrics. Today it has a staff of 51 psychiatrists, five psychologists, and four psychiatric social workers.

Throughout the years, there have been some leading principles which we have tried to keep in mind. Despite their seeming simplicity, these principles have been significant in our teaching and some of them are worth mentioning here.

The complexity of the theory which underlies and sustains our specialty often leads, in the course of our work, to a vagueness of concept. These must be systematically redefined and clarified in our minds. One of the major responsibilities of a teacher is constant restatement of his concepts in as clear and precise a form as possible. Only under these conditions can he teach well, comfortably, and without defensiveness.

[2]

Another factor may have equal importance, although this appears to be a truism also. In a general discussion of the process of teaching and learning, we would agree that the teacher has to take into account the conditions, expectations, and points of view that the student brings to any new field. This general principle becomes even more meaningful when we attempt to convey psychoanalytic concepts that are related to unconscious processes, and when the learning process is complicated by the orientation of doctors who are conditioned to expect tangible, measurable, and observable scientific facts. A genuine appreciation of the way in which the medically trained mind prefers to work has to be retained in our teaching. Only then can we communicate adequately in a form that bridges the difference between our respective fields. With it, we provide ourselves and the doctor with a basis for fuller participation in our particular system of thought and with an understanding of the use that can be made of it clinically.

It certainly is difficult to evaluate how essential such principles have proved to be because the process of adaption between our service and the rest of the hospital was gradual and almost imperceptible. Those who expected dramatic results overnight from such efforts may well have been disappointed. I believe that only a slow integration brings sound and lasting results. The concepts are too difficult and the process of comprehending is too subtle to be grasped quickly. Overenthusiasm in the beginning frequently leads to disappointment, and sometimes even to resentment of the unexpected difficulties which are inevitably encountered.

As our work progressed, we felt increasingly the need to broaden our knowledge and to reformulate our principles through exchange with a group of psychiatrists who were confronted with similar assignments and who have pursued similar goals for many years. Although we thought that such a meeting might be of interest to many, the replies to our invitations went far beyond our hopes. This response indicated how great an interest there is in sharing these problems, raising questions, and searching for solutions.

I am deeply grateful to those who have given their time and effort to this Symposium and who have come from all parts of the country to participate and contribute. I owe very special thanks to those members of my staff who took it upon themselves to help organize and execute this project which has outgrown all expectations. The Symposium Committee has borne the brunt of working out the endless complications: Doctors Henry G. Altman, Ralph J. Kahana, Arthur R. Kravitz, Cavin P. Leeman, John Vorenberg, and Norman E. Zinberg. I am grateful both to the members of their families and to their friends who lent their help so generously, as well as to the many volunteers not only from our own hospital but also from the Massachusetts Mental Health Center. I reserve a special gratitude for my secretary, Miriam Scheinfeldt, who patiently tended to the innumerable details. It is this combined effort which has made the project into an event that has not only provided us with a most satisfactory professional meeting, but also with an unusually pleasurable and gracious gathering of friends and colleagues.

When I came to edit this book, a rather unfamiliar task for me, I received invaluable support from Mrs. Harriet H. Gibney, who assisted me and introduced me to the secrets of the professional editor.

Grete L. Bibring, M.D.
Cambridge, Massachusetts

December, 1965

Can Psychiatry Be Taught?

Grete L. Bibring, M.D.

T HE TITLE OF THIS PAPER has elicited a variety of reactions, and I would like to share with you the motives underlying my choice. The question this topic poses is one which has intermittently preoccupied me throughout the years I have spent in teaching psychoanalytic psychiatry. The students with whom I have worked comprise a wide spectrum: candidates in training for psychoanalysis, medical colleagues learning to apply psychoanalytic psychology in their profession, students preparing for their work with patients, and psychiatric residents seeking improvement of their competence as therapists or as teachers.

Whether or not psychiatry can be taught is a genuine question. As a teacher I raised it when I had a feeling of disappointment, but even more so when I had a feeling of success. It concerned me not so much when I was observing the students of psychiatry in their attempts to learn, as it did during

[5]

my deliberations about the direction to be taken when setting out to teach a new course or when preparing to instruct a group of students in a different field.

With regard to the answers which I shall propose, however, they are quite tentative and quite personal and, as far as I am concerned, are still by no means satisfactory. The need for an exchange of ideas was the main motive underlying my decision to put the paper on our agenda and to invite the participants to join me in a search for further solutions. Because the history of teaching psychiatry suggests that answers have yet to be found—not only for the sake of those who want to benefit from learning, but for our own sake as well—we must clarify the field of our effort after many years of trial and error.

Thirty-five years ago Dr. Macfie Campbell (1930), then professor of psychiatry at Harvard Medical School and head of the Boston Psychopathic Hospital, delivered an address to a group of medical students at the opening of the New York Psychiatric Institute and Hospital, in an attempt to evoke their interest in his discipline. He indicated the difficulties one encounters and pointed out that the medical profession had not yet accepted the fact that psychiatry was changing. It was no longer the exclusive domain of psychiatrists with administrative talents working in hospitals with a huge aggregation of mentally disordered patients. The situation had been transformed and was now open to doctors with clinical and research interests in the topic of human maladjustment. Moreover, the speaker decried the fact that no premedical, basic preparation for psychiatry was given the students as compared with their background training in general medicine, and the fact that the medical schools make no adequate provisions for a satisfactory introduction to psychiatry. It thus becomes the

[6]

student's responsibility to make up for this gap in his training as best he can. Dr. Campbell spoke about the significance of psychotherapy for the physician who is not specifically interested in psychiatry or who does not feel confident enough in this area to pursue it as his specialty. He also stated that because every physician deals with problems of human nature he must not do so in a negligent or trifling way. To combat this state of affairs the schools and the hospitals would have to see to it that every physician who passes through such an institution has learned as an essential part of his professional duty how to recognize and deal more adequately with the patient himself, not only with his disease.

Since then many changes have taken place. Medical schools have set up curricula, colleges have introduced preparatory courses on normal and abnormal psychology, hospitals have established psychiatric units, departments, services. Yet when we listen to centenary and presidential addresses delivered by medical educators and leading physicians (George Packer Berry [1958], Lester Evans [1963], Alan Gregg [1948], Robert Loeb [1963], Sir George Pickering [1963]), when we follow the literature in journals of medical education, it seems as if the plea still goes on almost without change, as if we stood where we were 35 years ago, still convinced that psychiatry ought to be both taught and learned by physicians, and that something will have to be done about it. This somehow indicates that too little has been achieved, that the discipline has not found its proper place, and has not exerted its influence sufficiently. How can this be explained? It could be attributed to a variety of reasons: either the nature of the curricula does not allow sufficient time for it or it is not structured in the most adequate form; the teachers may be at fault, teaching either too little or too much, or the wrong things, or using the wrong

[7]

method; it may be due to the subject itself, which cannot be taught for some reason or another and therefore cannot be learned; and finally, there may be a combination of all these factors leading to a vicious circle of negative feedbacks. I shall attempt now to focus on some of the peculiarities, some of the obstacles and antinomies which we encounter in our task, and on the methods which are at our disposal in dealing with our teaching assignment.

Once, among a group of colleagues engaged in specialties different from my own, we were discussing the learning of foreign languages. One of the group, a most accomplished and unusually gifted doctor, told us that he had acquired his rather fluent knowledge of German from a German chef when, as a high-school boy, he was employed as a dishwasher in a Boston restaurant. He then added with an amused, almost mischievous smile (at least this is how it impressed me), that in spite of this sound preparation he very nearly flunked his German exam in college. Continuing with this account, he related the special circumstances which had unsettled him on this occasion. The examiner had asked him not to translate the German text word by word, but to read the whole page carefully first, and then translate it. The student found himself incapable of doing so, and when the professor offered him another chance with a second page of the book, he again failed almost completely. At this point I asked curiously and quite spontaneously: "Was it Thomas Mann?" "How did you guess this?" my friend asked. "I did not guess," was my reply, "I inferred it." This somewhat superior statement provoked the appropriate reaction, the request that I should demonstrate the process of inference drawing. Not to be found deficient, I did my very best to meet this challenge and what I could retrieve of my thoughts runs as follows: "This is a highly intelligent and gifted man. In all probability he was a very promising youngster, from Boston, earning his living as a dishwasher—a classical combination for a scholarship at Harvard."[1] Then there was the question of the German text: a Harvard language exam would not use a mediocre writer but an important one. Was this responsible for the doctor's special, amused smile, instead of a wistful expression at the recollection of his failure? Perhaps there was something amusing and intriguing about the assignment? Moreover, why was he asked to read the whole page? Not to translate word by word seems an appropriate request in a first-rate institution of higher learning, but why a whole page, why not just sentence by sentence? And at this moment, an idea, a recollection, an image emerged in my mind: what writer of first-rate standing, comparable to that of a first-rate college, would write sentences that are a page long? Then my question took shape: "Was it Thomas Mann?"

"Is this the way psychoanalysts think when they are on a job?" I was asked. With caution, I confirmed that it was, but I kept wondering whether this way of thinking is really so different from the way these doctors were thinking themselves, or whether we only utilize our thinking differently from the way they do? Does this difference then lead to some of our frequent misunderstandings and disagreements, and would better insights into these two positions help bridge the gap between us?

Let me quote here a passage pertaining to these questions, which has been excerpted from a piece of great literature:

[1] I hope it will be understood that our innermost thoughts frequently have this unequivocal directness which when said aloud or seen in print acquires a quality of irreverent or jocular unconcern.

[9]

One of the articles had a pencil mark at the heading, and I naturally began to run my eye through it. Its somewhat ambitious title was "The Book of Life," and it attempted to show how much an observant man might learn by an accurate and systematic examination of all that came his way. It struck me as being a remarkable mixture of shrewdness and absurdity. The reasoning was close and intense, but the deductions appeared to me to be far fetched and exaggerated. The writer claimed by a momentary expression, a twitch of a muscle or a glance of an eye, to fathom a man's inmost thoughts. Deceit, according to him, was an impossibility in the case of one trained to observation and analysis. His conclusions were as infallible as so many propositions of Euclid. So startling would his results appear to the uninitiated that until they learned the processes by which he had arrived at them they might well consider him a necromancer....

Like all other arts, the Science of Deduction and Analysis is one which can only be acquired by long and patient study, nor is life long enough to allow any mortal to attain the highest possible perfection in it. Before turning to those moral and mental aspects of the matter which present the greatest difficulties, let the inquirer begin by mastering more elementary problems. Let him, on meeting a fellow-mortal, learn at a glance to distinguish the history of the man, and the trade or profession to which he belongs. Puerile as such an exercise may seem, it sharpens the faculties of observation, and teaches one where to look and what to look for. By a man's fingernails, by his coat-sleeve, by his boots, by his trouser-knees, by the callosities of his forefinger and thumb, by his expression, by his shirtcuffs—by each of these things a man's calling is plainly revealed. That all united should fail to enlighten the competent inquirer is almost inconceivable.

"What ineffable twaddle!" I cried, slapping the magazine down on the table; "I never read such rubbish in my life."

"What is it?" asked Sherlock Holmes.

"Why, this article," I said, pointing at it with my egg-spoon as I sat down to my breakfast. "I see that you have read it, since you have marked it. I don't deny that it is smartly written. It irritates me, though. It is evidently the theory of some armchair lounger who evolves all these neat little paradoxes in the seclusion of his own study. It is not practical. I should like to see him clapped down in a third-class carriage on the underground, and asked to give the trades of all his fellow-travellers. I would lay a thousand to one against him."

"You would lose your money," Holmes remarked calmly. "As for the article, I wrote it myself."

"You!" (exclaimed Watson).

I hope you do not mind that I let Conan Doyle (1930, pp. 12-13) speak for me, especially since this imaginative author and physician created the hero of these tales in the image of his medical teacher, Dr. Joseph Bell of the Edinburgh Infirmary. Dr. Bell's diagnostic ability or "intuition" was famous and used to startle his students and colleagues (Doyle, Morley, 1930, p. x).

Having read to you Sherlock Holmes's credo, let us now study his relationship to his friend and (as he often calls him) partner Watson. In the beginning of their relationship, and in short fits of insight all through the years, Watson seems to have been a reasonably intelligent man who approached his friend Sherlock Holmes with a keenly analytic and discriminating mind, giving credit to his outstanding ability but also being fully capable of judging his great weaknesses, such as

[11]

his conceit, his showmanship, his domineering tendency, his addiction to success, and his biting, arrogant criticism of everyone else in his profession. When Sherlock Holmes reacted to Watson's admiring praise of his conclusions with the false modesty of his famous "Elementary!" or "Commonplace!" he conveyed clearly that his feat was elementary and commonplace only for him, the man who knew all the answers, but not for other mortals—including Watson. Yet why, apart from these episodes of intelligent comprehension, did Watson seem so inept, so blundering, so limited in the field of detection, though he gave it all his attention over many years, working closely with the greatest of detectives?

Why can't he learn from Sherlock Holmes? Sherlock Holmes appears to be ready to teach him. He shares with Watson all his thoughts; he points out to Watson the appropriate folders from his immense collection of files needed to help with each special case. He keeps in his apartment and offers his partner a complete library of specialized studies—written by himself—on all the essential elements which represent his own background knowledge, such as works on footprints, on residual ashes from different kinds of tobacco, on lethal poisons, etc. He shares with Watson during and after every assignment, in logical sequence, all the data he uses in arriving both at his intermediate and his final conclusions. Why can Watson not learn? Or is it that Sherlock Holmes cannot teach? His mode of instruction approximates what is commonly used and found acceptable as a method of teaching: to demonstrate over and over again one's technique in action, to give all the pertinent data which lead to the satisfactory results, so that the student can master them, and to refer to blibiographies from which additional knowledge can be acquired. Is this sufficient in Sherlock Holmes's field, and what bearing does it have on our work?

To answer these questions we have to recognize and define more clearly the different aspects of teaching which, though they have more general implications, will be discussed here in terms of their specific role in the teaching of psychiatry (Bruner, 1963). I would suggest that a distinction be made between two forms of instruction which are habitually used as synonyms: (a) the teaching of content and (b) the teaching of attitudes, of modes of approach that seem appropriate, even essential, for a high quality of performance in our field. For this I prefer the term "teaching by education," in keeping with Alfred North Whitehead's (1929; 1951) definition of education as "learning the art of utilizing knowledge."

(a) The teaching of content. This relates to presenting the subject matter, the data and facts, the basic rules and principles of scientific methodology and of techniques as they serve diagnosis and therapy—the do's and don't's, so to speak; it includes the teaching of the theory, the conceptual framework which provides the structure for the otherwise unmanageable variety of disparate data. The system that best fulfills this function today is psychoanalytic personality theory. This interrelated group of concepts has proved its primary value for understanding the development of personality, and of human behavior, both normal and abnormal. It is the system whose explanatory constructs offer the widest coverage for otherwise incomprehensible phenomena. Although it has not answered all the questions, and although it has mute and vague areas, it is at the same time open to examination, improvement, or correction, as is any sound and useful theory.

Psychoanalytic theory should be taught as a whole, not fractioned, not partly replaced, not even camouflaged, albeit in a clear and usable form, omitting those elements which mainly serve the interest of scholars and experts. This no doubt puts an additional burden on the instructor, who has to explicate with great care the complex data in their logical arrangement. A saying ascribed to Louis Agassiz may well serve here. Agassiz advised his pupils, if they wanted to write an article, to write it three times, first for a children's book, second for a ladies' magazine, and only third in its final form for a professional journal. Such steps in clarifying our own concepts might very well enhance the impact of our teaching.

By no means should we then exclude the teaching of additional viewpoints, though they may be opposed to or involved in dispute with psychoanalysis. I believe this too belongs to good instruction; it permits the students to compare and to understand better what may be lacking and what each of the systems may contribute.

To summarize: the teaching of content is essentially directed toward offering information and combating ignorance, and it may even be improved by what seems at present to be the concern of a large group of psychologists—the development of the psychotechnology of learning (Mosel, 1964), and computer-aided teaching (Feuerzweig, *et al.,* 1964). Success in acquiring this knowledge will depend on the ability to comprehend, on memory, and to some extent on learning by rote.

(b) If we now turn to the other form of teaching, *education,* we will recognize that additional factors, some of them rather different, are at play. To teach these attitudes, the mode of approach or (according to Whitehead) the "art of utilizing one's knowledge" is one of the central issues which concern us in psychiatry. It is this issue predominantly which I wanted to pursue when I raised the initial question: can psychiatry be taught? And this is the area where Sherlock Holmes failed Watson so completely.

[14]

I approach this topic cautiously and haltingly, because there exists no clear-cut glossary of qualifications for the psychiatric profession. Yet in teaching we want to provide assistance in the development of those characteristics which are most pertinent, yet are not well defined. Furthermore, for me an even greater difficulty arises from a different angle: to discuss befitting attributes in one's area of work consequently introduces our own system of values; and this may lead to the impression that I have set myself up as a paragon of virtue who has achieved professional perfection. I can only state simply and honestly that this is not my intention.

In order to achieve a better understanding it may be helpful to isolate some of the more important, habitual dispositions which medical people especially carry with them to psychiatry and which in turn, if they persist in their original form, may well incapacitate the student for further learning. I shall not spend any time on a central difficulty, the resistance that stems from emotional conflicts and repression, which may block a student's ability and willingness to enter the field with intellectual freedom and curiosity. This point will be discussed elsewhere in the present Symposium. But there are other contradictions between medical and psychiatric ways of functioning which are of importance here, and which lead to serious questions.

(1) One question is asked persistently: can a physician adhere to the strict rigor of cause and effect that is medical science while still maintaining the open spirit of explanation needed in understanding and appreciating a life?

(2) A second question (Whitehorn, 1963) is of even greater import: where clarity is the ideal, can the physician embrace a profession that must live consistently with ambiguity? He has learned to pursue action vigorously in diagnosis as

well as in therapy, because more often than not the well-being of his patient depends on quick and determined procedures. Can he learn to wait for additional information which he cannot force because the patient is not yet ready to talk or even ready to know about certain things? Can he keep in abeyance what he has already heard, observed, and inferred, until the data take on a life of their own, so to speak, forming a pattern that seems meaningful to the doctor and sufficiently clear to be transmitted to the patient? (Erik H. Erikson [1959a] calls this the convergence of data.)

The difference between the two specialists—our tendency to include as many data as possible in order to arrive at fuller understanding, and to sift out what is needed at different points while retaining the rest of the material for later use or for corrections under the same free-floating attention, in contrast to the physician's tendency to arrive at a decision in the quickest and most effective way, discarding what has not proved specifically relevant and excluding everything that may be distracting and confusing—represents one of the great antinomies leading to opposite ways of actions. We psychiatrists must keep to our basic principle of approach, holding in abeyance as many details as possible—whether or not they seem relevant at the time—until the major problems can be solved. I wonder whether our best physicians have not preserved some of this same attitude in themselves from the time when they were less experienced and less proficient—and this to their own advantage as well as to that of their patients.

(3) Can the doctor be professional toward his patient and at the same time care in a personal and responsible way that signals his concern to a human being who is troubled?

(4) Can he be dispassionate in comprehending and explaining a patient's emotional problem while at the same time

the patient is attempting to involve him personally in a transference relationship?

These are some of the contradictory patterns which create problems and difficulties for any student of psychiatry. In addition to these there is one question that has significance in other areas of education as well as in our own, a question which constitutes a hazard to learning wherever it cannot be solved: can the student appreciate and accept that his teacher has a point of view and an attitude that the student can apply and use only when he has understood it fully and has made it his own?

What now are the methods by which we attempt to educate a student of psychiatry? How can we help him to develop fruitful, appropriate attitudes and work habits? How does he learn those aspects of a professional competence which cannot be expressed in any actuarial form?

The primary means by which we convey these messages are provided by personal contact between the student and an experienced instructor. The student must be given the opportunity to observe his teacher in action; he must be able to raise questions related to what he has observed, what he has not understood, and what he has found difficult to accept. These questions provide a sound beginning for the instructor's contribution to education. He can explain what seemed incomprehensible; he can answer the criticism by presenting the reasoning behind his actions, or he may accept reasonable criticism, indicating why it has validity. The student will then have to try his own hand in dealing with patients and report his experience back to the instructor for discussion. It is in the supervisory hour that the student is presented with the greatest opportunity to learn his instructor's ways of functioning. Supervision must never be applied as Sherlock

[17]

Holmes applied it to Watson, that is, by answering Watson's stumbling attempts to offer his opinion on the crime with a barrage of brilliant—though in his case even correct—solutions. Conan Doyle took care of this. He made it easy for Sherlock Holmes to be infallible, much easier than life makes it for us, the supervisors.

Quite apart from the fact that this would be a distressing experience for the student instead of an encouragement, the supervisor does not even have at his disposal the patient's material but only that of the student—or what the student sees and arranges as the material. This does not provide a really safe basis for final and authoritative statements by the teacher. It permits us, however, to show the student what one *might* understand from the data he has provided. This appropriate, tentative approach is not an exercise in virtue but an important principle, a method in our educational task: to convey to the student the respect for data which is as fundamental for us as it is for any other scientist, and as it must become for the student. Therefore, we bring to the student's attention the fact that this is valuable material but that it hardly *can* be complete. Our interpretations will have to be understood by him as being provisional and general in nature, and the student will have to take this into account as he weighs and contrasts his interpretations against ours. He will always be the person who is closer to the source of information than we are, and may therefore know more about the patient than we possibly can. Furthermore, not only will this factor have to be considered, but also both he and the instructor have to await the further development of the material—whether it will prove or disprove today's conclusions.

Here again we discover that this simple principle contains a variety of essential professional modes of conduct. It reveals the responsibility of the experienced psychiatrist to wait and observe the further development of the case before insisting (if ever he does) that his impression has been correct; it discloses a certain tolerance and respect for the opinion of others, an attitude which the student has to acquire or maintain, as the case may be, vis-à-vis his patient, in the same manner in which he experiences it in the instructor's attitude toward himself; it introduces a safeguard against the inclination of some students to accept blindly the teacher's point of view, a tendency which often leads to an equally blind effort to prove him right by collecting confirmatory data for the next supervisory meeting. Whereas, the discussion I have described invites the student to become a collaborator, an investigator in his own right, one whose function is to express his reaction to the instructor's viewpoint and to check it against further material of the patient. And finally the student can learn from this principle that errors are not a disgraceful sign of incompetence —neither for the teacher nor for the student—but rather they offer a most valuable opportunity to broaden our understanding. As a matter of fact, I believe that we learn less from successful therapeutic operations—in such instances we can rarely say with full conviction which of the things we did was responsible for the positive result—than we may learn from failures which often show us clearly what kind of mistake has been made.

All in all, I do believe that supervision is of more importance in the education of the student, for whom it provides the opportunity to learn, not through memorizing but through identification with an accomplished and respected teacher, than it is a direct contribution to the treatment of any one individual patient under discussion. I am fully aware that this is only one aspect of the role which supervision plays in the learning process. Beyond this, it supplements the still scanty experience of the beginner by the rich and varied observations the teacher can bring from his practice; it broadens the student's understanding when not only similar but also contrasting clinical problems are introduced by the instructor; it allows the clinical picture to be linked to theoretical concepts and serves to elucidate both; and last but not least it provides a protective security for the patient as well as for the responsible but still somewhat insecure therapist.

Every medical student, whatever his main professional allegiance, should have the experience during his course in psychiatry of carrying at least a small number of cases in psychotherapy under supervision. Limited as this experience may be, there is no substitute for its impact on the learning process, particularly in regard to the role it plays in providing a genuine comprehension of the reality of psychological phenomena.

I have attempted to present here some of my thinking on the teaching of psychoanalytic psychiatry, although I am quite sure that all of you have your own answers. I feel it is important to exchange our ideas, and even more important to put on record that this question must be left open until a satisfactory solution is found. This symposium has already shown how much interesting and constructive thinking can be assembled by merely announcing an inquiry.

We have learned the answers, all the answers:
It is the questions we do not know.

(Archibald MacLeish, 1952)

PANEL I: MEDICAL STUDENTS

Chairman, GRETE L. BIBRING

Psychoanalytic Teaching in the Medical School

Thomas F. Dwyer, M.D.

UNDER THIS BROAD TITLE my presentation concerns itself primarily with one issue: the scientific status of psychoanalysis today. I shall discuss how the scientific standing of psychoanalysis presents certain problems for the teaching of dynamic psychiatry, and shall examine some solutions for this problem. In emphasizing this subject I do not mean to belittle the importance of other difficulties in the teaching of dynamic psychiatry; it is my aim to focus on one problem that has perhaps not been given sufficient attention.

Experimentation and major changes in medical education have displayed a marked acceleration since World War II, and this trend of more frequent and sweeping reorganizations of the curriculum with regard to content and methods of teaching seems likely to continue. As the factors giving impetus to these changes are numerous, only two that are particularly relevant to today's presentation will be singled out

[23]

here: the explosion of discoveries in the sciences that are basic to medicine; the waxing and waning influence of psychoanalysis in the medical curriculum.

During the past two decades changes in teaching psychiatry to medical students have also been extensive, and further major experiments and alterations are clearly in sight. The reasons for some of the changes in the psychiatric curriculum require an historical perspective, which needs only a broad, sweeping treatment for this occasion; the details are well represented elsewhere (APA, 1952; APA, 1953; GAP, 1962).

Prior to World War II changes in psychiatric teaching were slow and few. Descriptive psychiatry, dealing predominantly with the psychoses, remained the core of psychiatric programs and gave way only gradually and incompletely to courses in psychobiology, which during the 1930's existed as perhaps the leading systematic presentation of psychiatry. Psychoanalytic concepts, introduced into medical education in a very few places in the 1930's, rapidly took a leading position in medical schools throughout this country during the 1940's and 1950's. During the same two latter decades, psychiatric teaching was for the first time given a major position in the preclinical curriculum of most medical schools, as exemplified by an increase on a national scale from an average of 20 hours during the first two years of medical school in 1940, to an average of 73 hours in 1960. During the 1950's there began further significant changes in psychiatric teaching with the introduction of courses by social psychologists, sociologists, anthropologists, and others, and with this development we are brought to the present period.

In a GAP Report published in October, 1962, the chapter on historical perspective ends as follows:

[24]

It would seem that certain expectations of psychiatric educators in earlier years failed to materialize. [First, academic psychology; second, psychobiology; and third, the psychosomatic and liaison services—each seemed promising in its turn, and then receded. Finally,] fourth, it seems to this Committee that some of the enthusiasm for integrating psychoanalytic concepts completely with psychiatric education—a prominent goal following World War II—has now leveled off.

The rapid expansion of psychoanalytic teaching needs to be examined, although no comprehensive explanation will be attempted here. On the negative side, the inadequacy of previous theories of human behavior, including psychobiology, had left a relative vacuum in the medical schools' curricula. On the positive side, the general excellence of the psychiatric training programs set up for the US Armed Forces during World War II, especially those programs led by Grinker, Kaufman, and Murray, gave a clear demonstration of the usefulness of applied psychoanalytic concepts in treating war neuroses. After the War, the Commonwealth Fund was one of the prime movers in supporting programs in medical schools to translate the wartime application of psychoanalytic concepts to civilian practice. In this same period, a number of psychoanalysts whose teaching efforts had been largely devoted to psychoanalytic institutes began teaching in the university general hospital and in the medical schools, as a result of which psychoanalysis was brought closer to the main stream of medicine.

It has been in this encounter with the general practice of medicine that psychoanalysis has made one of its most significant and lasting contributions to the teaching of the medical student. Psychoanalytic constructs "straight from the couch" do not, to understate the point, catch the attention and interest of the medical student and physician. In contrast, psychoanalytic concepts translated in response to the exigencies of medical practice, have been outstandingly useful. By way of brief example: a psychiatric instructor who discusses with his surgical colleague a patient's castration anxiety will usually have lost his audience in brief order; the psychiatrist, however, who describes the same patient as a person excessively afraid of passivity and of being attacked, especially by means of surgical procedures, with the possible development of persecutory ideas in the postoperative period, will more often than not find himself working with a surgeon who is willing to postpone an operation, allowing the time to deal with the acute emotional problems. Many other psychoanalytic concepts translated appropriately, that is, into a language which is meaningful and useful to the practicing physician while not compromising any of the original psychoanalytic insight, have succeeded in becoming what appears to be a permanent part of medical education. What is referred to here are such things as the teaching of basic techniques in human interaction between physician and patient. In this area information coming originally from psychoanalysis—now much modified for application in medical practice—has become so accepted a part of medical education that, at least in some quarters, it is hardly questioned. The fact that such teaching is no longer usually labeled psychoanalytic may account for some of the apparent waning of psychoanalytic teaching in the medical schools today.

The shrinking of psychoanalytic teaching in the medical curriculum is, however, not only apparent but also real. In at least a few medical schools psychoanalytic teaching reached a peak in the mid-50's, leveled off during the next five years, and in the past several years has shown some initially small but significant losses. One emerging pattern of change is that the behavioral sciences already mentioned (anthropology, sociology, and others) are beginning to displace some of the analytic teaching, especially during the first year. The avowed aims of such changes—for example, to broaden the base of the student's understanding of human behavior, to make the teaching rest on more "scientific" observations, to avoid the student's becoming prematurely committed to any "unproven" set of hypotheses—are always estimable, but the effect of such courses can be abysmal. The medical student typically catches only brief glimpses of one or another of the behavioral sciences. The material contained therein generally does not permit of assimilation into the larger body of his medical education, and, more seriously, he is likely to get an inadequate picture of human development from the viewpoint of dynamic psychology.

Why this retrenchment in the number of hours available for teaching dynamic psychiatry, actual in the examples I have just cited and imminent in a number of other medical schools where psychoanalytic teaching and principles are being questioned more sharply than has been the case for a couple of decades? What is the scientific standing of psychoanalysis in the 1960's—that is, in a period when the first-year medical student is likely to be more familiar with the submolecular structure of the cell than he is with the picture revealed by the conventional microscope? Has psychoanalytic research, in its own way, maintained some degree of progression comparable to research in other medical sciences? If one reviews the psychoanalytic literature, one is forced to conclude that adequate research into those psychoanalytic theories that can be investigated by methods other than by psychoanalysis itself—research aiming at a verifiable body of data capable of being communicated to other scientists by the usual modes, that is, without "faith"—has been very slow in developing.

This lag in appropriate psychoanalytic research was deplored as early as 1952 by Glover, who noted an increasing tendency on the part of psychoanalysts to neglect applying to their data such scientific controls as were available. Collaborative investigations by psychoanalysts and other scientists have made contributions to one or the other field and on occasion have added significant discoveries. There continues, however, too much guardedness in most encounters between psychoanalysts and other behavioral scientists. Although there are happily an increasing number of exceptions, many behavioral scientists from outside the field of psychoanalysis approach psychoanalysts as though the latter were antiscientific members of a cult, espousing a set of doctrines which have had to be accepted without examination, usually during the process of a personal psychoanalysis. Unfortunately this biased picture, which amounts to a caricature if applied to all psychoanalysts, is an accurate representation of a few. In addition, a number of psychoanalysts, while not fitting the stereotype, do at times adopt some of the attitudes and concepts of the stereotype, especially when on the defensive.

Equally as often, other behavioral scientists are guilty of irrationality in their response, for example, by insisting that a statistical proof be adduced for a psychoanalytic theory where this may be irrelevant or impossible. Clearly, the time is long overdue for the end of this bickering, and there are already examples of fruitful, cooperative efforts between psychoanalysts and other social-behavioral scientists.

The impact of some of the problems that have been part

of psychoanalytic research on the teaching of dynamic psychiatry was forecast in the 1951 Conference on Psychiatry and Medical Education (APA, 1952). In the book reporting this conference the shortest chapter is entitled, "The Scientific Foundations of Psychiatry." It discusses the futile attempts made at this conference to agree upon working principles as a basis for systematic, undergraduate instruction in psychiatry not to mention the dismaying lack of agreement on the basic principles of "psychodynamics." In the final analysis only a hope remained:

> There can be little question as to the propriety and the need for such research activities (testing out psychodynamic theory in humans, in a clinical setting and in animal studies) in the department responsible for basic teaching in psychodynamics; otherwise teaching degenerates into mere indoctrination.

It was felt that the following conference, to be held in 1952, would have a "greater measure of success" in clarifying and formulating the scientific foundations of psychiatry.

The findings of the 1952 Conference, reported in *The Psychiatrist: His Training and Development* (APA, 1953), especially as recorded in the chapter entitled "Psychodynamics," are instructive: general agreement was reached on one basic proposition, "that psychodynamics is concerned with understanding the motives of human behavior." It was further agreed broadly that an understanding of motivation appeared to form the basis of a sound, rational practice as applied to psychotherapy or psychopathology. Beyond these points of agreement, the conference found itself in greater disagreement than agreement with regard to motivational theories.

[29]

This dissension that has existed among many who practice psychoanalysis or who have worked with psychodynamic principles, as well as the continued aversion to psychodynamics expressed by others, can no longer be explained simply on the basis of such factors as emotional resistance to the subject matter. Personal and emotional responses continue to contribute to the disputes that exist in the field. However, at this stage in the history of psychoanalysis it is necessary to take note of the extent to which the disagreements have been supported, until quite recently, by the relative paucity of efforts to rescue psychoanalytic theory from the realm of "private" opinion and to channel it into the arena of "public" understanding—that is, we must seek ways to produce data capable of being transmitted with their proof from one psychoanalyst to another scientist.

This is not an invitation for psychoanalysts (or for other scientists who might work with them) to conclude that unless psychoanalysis imitates the physical sciences in its methods of investigation it is not a science. Many of the decisive proofs in the physical sciences have been achieved precisely because what was being investigated was capable of being manipulated under exactly those circumstances in which all essential variables except the one under investigation could be kept constant, thus allowing for a relatively exact proof (or disproof) of that hypothesis being investigated. Many important discoveries that can contribute to the science of human behavior are being made and will be made by this kind of scientific approach. However, it appears logically impossible that all human behavior will ever lend itself to "scientific" explanation, if we hold to the narrow view that a hypothesis cannot be proven or disproven unless it can be tested in a laboratory or its equivalent. Investigations into human behavior can and should include experimental studies (for example, testing some of the theories about the emotional significance of mouth activities as manifested in the normal infant's sucking response in comparison to that of the infant born with a cleft palate); but such experimental studies will rarely, if ever, have the precision, the exactitude of proof, of the usual experimental studies in the physical sciences. We must therefore depend largely on careful observation—and "careful" in this context means less dependence on that kind of contribution by individual investigators which reports one case or a series of cases, and in which each investigator reports his own observations and his own conclusions. As valuable as these contributions will always remain in terms of increasing our understanding in human psychology of what may be true, they must be supplemented, more than has been done until now, by other methods in which, for example, groups of investigators working together on the very propositions forwarded by individual investigators, in carefully designed studies, test various hypotheses of human behavior much more rigorously than is usually possible by one individual.

These remarks are not intended to imply any sacred quality about groups of investigators, nor are they intended to deny the obvious, namely, that new ideas will continue to arise in the mind of the individual scientist. Nevertheless, in this stage of the development of psychoanalysis, major steps need to be taken by investigators who understand psychoanalysis, who can work together, and who can devote themselves, not to system-building, but to lessening the confusion of tongues in the house of psychoanalysis before the latter begins to speak authoritatively to other sciences. A careful individual psychoanalysis can be a much more scientifi-

[31]

THOMAS F. DWYER

cally controlled investigation of behavior than any of the most carefully designed projects dreamed up by the wildest detractors of psychoanalysis—but this should not be enough for psychoanalysts. Science requires proof as well as communicability; it is in this latter area that psychoanalysis has until the recent past performed so poorly.

Fortunately, at the time that the 1951 and 1952 conferences were reported, psychoanalytic research projects were already being initiated (and more have since been started) which are making it possible to fulfill the promise that certain aspects of psychoanalytic theory can at least be studied by methods that are familiar or explicable to other scientists. It seems significant that most of these new developments in research and psychoanalysis have taken place in medical settings where one of the more obvious pressures on the psychoanalytic investigator is to communicate to medical colleagues who are not psychoanalysts. Time permits the naming of only a few of the types of researches that are referred to here: the work of the late Ernst Kris and his collaborators at Yale; the project known as the Hampstead Index (Sandler, 1962) in London; and the study of pregnancy carried out in Boston under the leadership of Grete L. Bibring (1959; 1961). By now many other comparable studies are being carried out, signaling a new spirit of scientific inquiry well-exemplified by the writings of John Benjamin. We can now confidently anticipate in the coming years substantial contributions to the psychoanalytic science of psychology—contributions both useful in furthering the treatment of ill humans and effective in promoting what can be taught.

The fact must be faced, however, that even with the most careful research, it is unlikely that the demonstration of principles about human behavior will ever be as conclusive as the proof or the disproof of a hypothesis in the physical sciences. It is exceedingly important that this concept be clear in our minds, and that in turn such differences as inevitably exist in a science of human behavior be made increasingly explicit by the investigator and for the student.

Meanwhile, what can be taught? And how and when should it be taught? One way to respond to the recognition of where dynamic psychiatry stands as a science is to postpone teaching this subject until the student has begun to have a more intensive contact with patients. There are, I believe, weighty arguments against this. It can be argued that one year is not too much time for the student to devote himself exclusively to the basic medical sciences, so that he may, one hopes, become imbued with the scientific method and thereafter think as a scientist as well as a physician. One can only agree with the tenor of this argument. A problem arises, however, because the student during the course of a year is not simply being introduced to science—he is also being introduced to medicine. Since the subject matter of medicine is man, a totality more complicated than the sum of its parts, surely it is unnecessarily risky to subject the future physician to an entire year which implies, if it does not state, that man consists of a series of chemical and physical systems and can be totally understood in such terms. The student may or may not become more of a scientist after such a year, but there is a clear danger of his becoming the kind of "scientist" that forms a stereotype in the minds of many a lay person, and which has some basis in reality, namely, a person who is overly preoccupied with narrow interests and knowledge at the expense of a broader awareness of the human who is sick.

These remarks may sound antiscientific, when indeed they are intended only to emphasize a truism: that the practicing physician should be more than a scientist. Certainly the needs in the undergraduate curriculum for the teaching of the so-called hard sciences can only increase, but this should not be at the expense of the total exclusion of instruction that adequately keeps the human being on stage while his parts are being played out in various courses. How to keep the human being before the student, especially during the first two years will remain the subject for debate. (I shall show my own preference on this subject shortly.) Home Care Programs, assigning the student to a family, etc., are justifiably criticized when such programs have miscarried and have thereby placed the emphasis on premature medical practice rather than on helping the student to maintain an image of the whole human being concomitant with his observations of human parts in the laboratory.

With regard to the role of dynamic psychiatry in assisting the student in his view of the total human, one is prompted to ask: if that which can be presented in the first years cannot emulate the teaching in the other medical courses, what can be done besides abandoning such teaching? There is an approach to the teaching of human behavior which should be employed during the first years—an approach which, instead of retreating before the differences between the science of human behavior and the other sciences, takes advantage of these differences and capitalizes on the human experiences of the student up to the time that he enters medical school. This style of teaching recognizes that, in contrast to the student's premedical preparation for advanced courses in other areas, he has not had, and cannot now have, comparable preparatory courses in "Behavior I," "Behavior II," etc. However, it cannot be ignored that the student has already lived approximately 20 years as an infant, a child, an adolescent, and a young adult; usually he is a brother or a sister, a son or daughter; and finally, he has had various interactions with parents, authorities, peers, etc. In other words, the student has had experiences, unique in each case, but certainly containing some universals that can be extracted to effect a more systematic study of human behavior than he has had occasion to develop on his own in living as a social animal. To exploit these experiences for further learning means that the teaching of human behavior, especially in the first and second years in medical school, should center on patients who are for the most part psychologically normal (but who are undergoing stress of one kind or another, if only as a result of their physical illness, because under stress the psychological mechanisms are so greatly highlighted). This teaching would explicate that which is universal among the patients' various responses, and at the same time would resonate that which is universal among the students' past experiences, comparable to what they are seeing in their patients.

The approach described requires that small groups of students meet weekly with one or two psychiatric instructors (over a period of months, beginning in the first year) and that they concentrate (in that year especially) on the normal in human psychological development and behavior.

What needs to be taught and can be taught here? Only examples can be given, not an all-inclusive program: (1) the existence and workings of normal psychological defense processes, whose importance can hardly be argued any longer by any honest and serious investigator of human behavior; (2) the existence of relatively stable behavioral equilibria in adults—that is, broad patterns of response which are predictable for each individual in that they repeat themselves, not in detailed fashion, but in the gross yet significant scheme of

[35]

behavioral response for any individual in one stress situation after another, no matter how different the types of stress may be. Such teaching would provide the basis for later courses in psychopathology in the second and subsequent years, in which the dynamics of the neuroses and psychoses would be taught in addition to examination of other explanations for mental disturbance.

In the broadest sense, what is at stake here is not only a more effective teaching of psychiatry to medical students, but also the urgent need for dynamic psychiatry to fill a vital part of the students' training to become physicians. There is no need to reiterate the immense benefits that followed the establishment of scientific medicine in our schools during the early decades of this century. The inclusion of more and more "hard" science in the medical curriculum is going to continue, and those concerned with the future of medicine welcome this fact. Yet, great as the gains to medicine from such teaching have been, there have been some negative results too, and an examination of these latter results—as well as the attempts to nullify them—should not be considered antiscientific (Chapman, 1956). Misunderstood and misapplied as the "Art of Medicine" and the "Whole Patient" have been at times, the fact is that our modern medical schools have graduated and are graduating some doctors who, as practicing physicians, do not deal adequately with the human beings who present themselves for medical care. The unfortunate state of fragmentation existing in current medical practice is surely not due to the teaching of science in medical schools, nor does the cure lie in the reduction of scientific courses. The need is for a counterbalancing force during the medical student's education, a force that is not antiscientific (and may even be scientific in a different way from a minute and necessary attention to systems, cells, and molecules), a force that will not let the student forget during his school years or afterwards that he is always dealing with the entire human organism as well as with the parts of that organism.

To summarize briefly: an attempt has been made to assess the role that psychodynamic concepts have been playing and will continue to play in undergraduate medical education, against a background of the relatively sweeping changes in medical education itself. Attention has been paid to some of the continuing problems that exist in the teaching of dynamic psychiatry, especially those problems that arise from the need for an increase in certain kinds of research in the field of psychoanalysis. Finally, I have expressed some opinions as to the increasing importance of the teaching of dynamic psychiatry throughout the undergraduate medical years, in response to other changes in medical education.

Teaching Dynamic Psychiatry to Medical Students

CHARLES W. TIDD, M.D.

In thinking about the question, "Can Psychiatry Be Taught?" my first response was, "Yes, given certain conditions." A primary and practical consideration in this regard concerns who has the authority to say what *may* be taught in a medical school or hospital. Closely connected with this concern is another: Just what is meant by "psychiatry?" Fortunately, we have been asked to consider a more specific question in that we have narrowed our subject to dynamic psychiatry. But before examining this area I should like to go back to the matter of administrative authority and remind you that it was not many years ago that the question of whether psychiatry could be taught might have been, and in some cases was, answered in the negative at the administrative level. Typically the question of what was involved in the definition or content of psychiatry was important, especially when psychoanalytic ideas were first introduced. There is no point in reviewing the historical details of the conflict between those who backed dynamic ideas and those who were content with a descriptive or organic approach, except to remind ourselves that this was a very real problem and that the people involved were affected in important ways. It is my contention that the parties to this controversy continue to be affected in varying degrees, and that the conflict continues, although its manifestations are different. I will expand upon this later in discussing some current problems in teaching.

In asking the question, "Can dynamic psychiatry be taught to medical students?" there is an implied emphasis on the subject, "dynamic psychiatry," suggesting that there may be something in the nature of the subject which might interfere or prevent its being taught or learned. Although I reject such a notion, along with many others engaged in this effort, I most willingly admit that there are special problems in attempting to teach dynamic psychiatry.

This brings me to the second part of the title of our symposium: "A reappraisal of the goals and techniques of the teaching of psychiatry." It happens that this meeting was announced at about the same time I suggested that a workshop be set up at the meeting of the American Psychoanalytic Association on practically the same subject. Judging from the response to this meeting and to the workshop which was held in May 1964, I think it is quite evident that many people are interested in getting together to talk things over. We are here then to take a good hard look at what we have been doing and to consider possibilities and proposals for change.

Historical accounts of the teaching of dynamic psychiatry to medical students have been presented by a number of people. Freud (1919) discussed the teaching of psychoanalysis in universities and in medical schools, and expressed the idea that

[39]

the student would not learn "psychoanalysis proper," but that "it will be enough if he learns something *about* psychoanalysis and something from it." Since World War II, S. Szurek (1957), G. Ham (1961), C. W. Tidd (1960), and others have reported on the subject.

In addition, the reports of the Ithaca Conference in 1951-1952 (APA, 1952, 1953) provided definitions and established certain basic principles regarding the teaching of dynamic psychiatry in medical schools. There have also been reports from other committees on the subject (GAP, 1948; GAP, 1958; APA, 1956; GAP, 1962). These papers and reports show that before World War II there were only a few instances in which serious attempts were made to introduce dynamic psychiatry into the medical curriculum. Immediately following the war, however, the subject came to be included in the curriculum of most medical schools in the United States, as a result of the rapid growth of the movement.

In the May 1964 workshop on teaching psychoanalytic concepts to medical students, papers were presented by Drs. Stoller, Brosin, Michaels, and Harper.[1] Dr. Joseph Natterson, who was a participant, also served as a recorder, and I have drawn on his report for ideas expressed in the workshop. Dr. Stoller opened the discussion with a paper, "Impediments to Teaching Psychoanalytic Concepts to Medical Students," which expressed the idea that the question of whether or not psychoanalytic concepts can be taught is a rhetorical one, since these concepts have been taught for some years. He stated that "the real problem is not whether psychoanalytic concepts can be taught but whether they can be taught in such a way that they

[1] Unpublished transactions of the workshop of the American Psychoanalytic Association, held at the annual meeting, Los Angeles, May, 1964.

[40]

can be learned." The point was made that teaching skill is of utmost importance; in its absence the teacher's knowledge, wisdom, intelligence, or ability as a psychoanalyst is to little or no avail. Dr. Stoller maintained that psychoanalytic concepts can be effectively derived from observable data and that they can be taught along with other behavioral science material. He also pointed out that for the past 15 years many psychoanalyst-teachers have had carte blanche in undergraduate teaching, but that the situation is changing, particularly with regard to preclinical teaching, and that psychoanalysts must make changes where necessary.

Dr. Brosin emphasized the need to plan and prepare for changes in approach, claiming that there is much to be done to clarify and define concepts and to improve teaching techniques. He advocated that we must strive for a comprehensive theory of human behavior, and stressed the importance of integrating the behavioral sciences with psychoanalytic teaching.

Dr. Michaels "emphasized psychoanalysis as a psychology rather than 'just' a medical discipline, preferring to regard psychoanalysis as a general system of psychology rather than seeing psychiatry as a part of behavioral science." He then referred to the reports of the Committee on the Teaching of Psychoanalysis in Medical Schools (established in 1948 under the direction of Dr. Grete L. Bibring) to the American Psychoanalytic Association. The Committee recommended that students be taught to "handle patients with medical problems to promote maximum understanding with a minimum of therapeutic activity" (quoting Dr. Bibring). Dr. Michaels also noted that "in point of view, then, the student automatically assumes the relevance of the psychiatric approach."

Dr. Harper continued the discussion by expressing the idea

[41]

that "most medical students want to become good doctors, but medical schools have dampened students' enthusiasm for understanding people, partly by the prevailing emphasis on severe skepticism. Thus the student comes to expect similar skepticism of his psychoanalyst instructors. Although psychoanalysis is a 'soft' science, the analyst need not be apologetic since he has a subtle, useful system." He described the integrated program at Western Reserve to illustrate the ways in which that institution has attempted to deal with the problems of teaching dynamic psychiatry. Later in this paper I will report other ideas which were expressed at the workshop.

To summarize the history, we can say that after World War II there appeared an increasing number of opportunities for psychoanalytically trained people to teach in medical schools. It is certain that the quality of such teaching has varied considerably and that the results have been similarly uneven. With an increasing amount of experience, and with the clarification of the wide range of problems involved in teaching, many teachers are interested in studying what has been done and in trying to find better ways to accomplish the task. In the following material I shall discuss the subject of goals, students and teachers, what is to be taught, and some proposed methods of teaching it.

In considering the question of goals in teaching dynamic psychiatry to medical students, I would like to begin by examining the overall aim of the medical curriculum as a whole. Essentially this goal is to give the student as advantageous a start as is possible on the road to becoming a good physician. As teachers of psychiatry we have constantly to bear in mind the student's entire program when planning the instruction in psychiatry. Anyone who has sat in on the meetings of a curriculum committee knows that from a practical point of view it is impossible to do otherwise. Our goal as teachers of dynamic psychiatry then is to provide the medical student with information which will lead him to a comprehensive understanding of the mental and emotional elements of human personality and human illness.

Having stated the goal, let us turn our attention to the ways by which it may be achieved through a consideration of the people who are trying to learn. On the basis of the candidates selected by the admissions committee, we can make several statements. Chronologically, most of them are young adults but, according to Stoller (reported at the May, 1964 workshop), as a group they appear to be less well developed emotionally than many other individuals in the same age group.

On starting medical school, our students, for the greater part, are still adolescent. In certain areas of their lives, by a survival of those most fit to get through medical school, they have not finished with many adolescent problems which many their age have resolved. By elaborating their intellectual defenses, they not only can postpone their confrontation with maturity but can also put this to good stead in delaying identity formation, i.e., they have the capacity to continue being students and therefore to continue to be dependent long after they are biologically equipped for a more definitive identity. First, simply because they are adolescent, and second, because they must make sure of a defense to prolong their adolescence, they are still in the midst of unfinished struggles against instinctual forces. The latter are undoubtedly the enemies of a successful studentship. Therefore, as adolescents would feel if permitted to free-associate, our students must acquire insight into these forces as a threat. Such insight may then be avoided by such defense mechanisms as denial, scorn, total intellectual acceptance, sleepiness, etc.

While I am concerned about the fact that many (or most) students continue to function in a strongly dependent position over an extended number of years, I believe Dr. Stoller has overemphasized the degree of adolescence. I have been impressed with the first-year medical students' ability to approach the study of medicine with much eagerness and enthusiasm. Most of these people have finished four years of university work and are still able to begin this new undertaking with freshness and vigor.

A large number of the incoming students have had limited life experiences, and this is of importance in the attempt to teach them dynamic concepts. Closely related is the important matter of their premedical training. In spite of the fact that some medical schools have publicly announced that they no longer require marked emphasis on science courses in the premedical work and that they welcome students with majors in the humanities, most students do continue to choose science. I have heard students say that having been accepted for medical school, they then took the courses in college that they "liked," meaning courses in the humanities.

The first-year medical students are intelligent young people who have been selected largely on the basis of intellectual achievement, with special emphasis on their work in the sciences. Few of them have had as much work in the humanities and social sciences as the teacher of dynamic psychiatry would hopefully anticipate; some have strong biases and prejudices which tend to interfere with their learning of psychodynamics. On the other hand, there are those whose interest in human behavior facilitates their ability to learn quickly. Thus there is a rather wide range represented—at one end is the "natural" and at the other the "impossible." It is with this in mind that I shall later emphasize what I believe to be of crucial importance in the attempt to teach dynamic psychiatry, namely, that these individual differences should be taken into account as much as possible.

The question of resistance in medical students is one which has elicited much consideration and discussion. As is true of other variables, there are individual differences in the responses of the students. The teacher attempts to present psychoanalytic concepts to the students so that these ideas will serve as a basis for understanding the behavior of patients. In this attempt the student is asked to take his own feelings into account, either directly or indirectly. No analyst should be surprised to see evidence of resistance when this attempt is made. The question of how much resistance should be dealt with is not an easy one. It is important to keep this factor of resistance in mind throughout all aspects of the teaching situation, starting with the plans for setting up a program. I believe that if one arranges the presentation of material over the four-year period, keeping a sharp eye to both sequence and continuity, as well as maturation of the student, this will help to solve the problem of resistance. There is generally an impressive degree of maturation from year to year in most students, and with it one sees an increased capacity to accept fundamental concepts, a capacity which it is important to utilize.

And now to turn to the other person who is principally involved in the teaching-learning situation, the teacher. Again it is helpful to look briefly at the history. Before World War II the usual situation was that all psychiatry courses were taught in conjunction with neurology in a department of neurology or one of neurology and psychiatry. The formal training of many of the teachers had been primarily in neurology. There were exceptions, but certainly there was no question as to who had the administrative authority. During and after the war this changed abruptly, so that the psychoanalytically trained psychiatrist had many more opportunities to teach in medical schools. Without attempting to catalogue the accomplishments or failures of the past 20 years, I think we can summarize some of the results of this experience as it concerns the teacher of dynamic psychiatry. Again, it has been shown that some people have talent as teachers. Given adequate talent, the person who has the interest and energy may learn and develop teaching skills. In the ideal situation, the teacher with talent and ability has the opportunity to meet and work with students who are bright and who want to learn.

There is another important factor in this teaching experience, one which cannot be ignored: the milieu of the medical school. By "milieu" I refer principally to the members of the faculty and their attitudes toward psychiatry. This includes members of the faculty within the department of psychiatry as well as those faculty members in the other departments. Here again the teacher of dynamic psychiatry has to take the factor of resistance into consideration. Other factors are important—ignorance, for example, and its close associates, bias and prejudice. These important forces must be seen as clearly as possible, and measures must be set up to deal with them.

During the past few years in most departments of psychiatry, if not all, considerable attention has been focused on the place of the behavioral sciences in the medical curriculum. A number of questions have been raised: should information from the behavioral sciences be included in the medical curriculum? Is it the responsibility of the department of psychiatry to see that such information is included? What material from which sciences should be used? If we assume that these decisions have been made in the affirmative, who will teach the material? These are important questions, and it certainly is understandable that psychiatrists are interested in them. However, it is also necessary that we consider these questions and their possible answers in close connection with the principal goal or goals of the psychiatric staff. The extremely important matter of available teaching time has to be considered. Assuming that it has been possible to select material which is considered relevant from anthropology, sociology, psychology, ethology, and other disciplines, and that one has teachers who are capable of presenting this material skillfully so that it can be integrated into the main body of dynamic psychiatry and the whole medical curriculum by the medical student, is the psychiatric staff justified in giving up the time required? When I speak of giving up time, I mean omitting part of the material which has previously been carefully selected and considered essential to the most effective presentation. In the case I have just cited, it has to do in most instances with material concerning psychosexual development which is used as a starting point, or foundation, for the entire four-year program. My own feeling is that relinquishing this time is not justified, unless one is able to find an effective means of presenting the psychosexual material in less time.

It is possible that such questions, discussions, and decisions occurring in a department of psychiatry *may* represent varying degrees of resistance to basic psychoanalytic concepts. On the other hand, there is no question but that many or most psychoanalysts interested in teaching are genuinely interested in utilizing material from these other disciplines. It is difficult to see how anyone could object to an ongoing attempt to build

[47]

a more comprehensive theoretical framework for the understanding of human behavior. It appears that the psychoanalytic model is the most promising both for the further development of psychoanalysis itself and for the inclusion of information from other sources.

The question of the effects which faculty members in other departments have on the teaching of dynamic psychiatry is one which does not lend itself to a simple and definitive answer. There is a wide range of attitudes, running from open antagonism to a sympathetic and informed acceptance. That these attitudes do affect the medical student is unquestionably true, but it is impossible to predict the degree to which he is affected or whether the effect will be positive or negative. Various suggestions have been made in the attempt to overcome those negative attitudes within the educational milieu which interfere with the student's acquisition of psychiatric knowledge. There is reason to believe that, given enough time and the opportunity for faculty members to get to know one another, some changes may be effected.

In general, however, it is a problem which will continue indefinitely, and one for which there are no set answers. The underlying fact that people try to avoid the perception and understanding of irrational behavior continues to be decisive. If one looks at the history of the treatment of mentally ill people, there is some evidence to suggest that this negative attitude has been true to a greater degree in medical people than in the general population. During the past 50 years there has been an emphasis on the development of the "science" of medicine in which the definition of science has been too narrow and restricted, as a result of which materials and phenomena which could not be measured by the methods of the physical sciences were dismissed in various ways. The attitude or response of the psychiatrist when confronted or opposed by negative elements in his colleagues may have a decisive effect on the medical student. It is not my intention, however, to recommend a particular attitude for all cases.

Up to this point we have considered the medical student, the teacher, and the milieu in which the students and teachers interact. Each of these areas will be open for further discussion later. Let us turn now to the questions of subject matter and methods of teaching. I shall start with the assumption that what we refer to as dynamic psychiatry is based principally on psychoanalytic concepts. Our task as teachers is to present those concepts to medical students who, with certain rare exceptions, have not had the experience of personal analysis and are not likely to have it during medical-school years.

I have already mentioned the importance of planning the instruction in psychiatry so that the work of all four years is considered as a whole. In this way not only is there a strong element of continuity, but also various elements may be added or repeated to fit in with the development and maturation of the student.

Most psychiatric programs are initiated in the first year of medical school, and I believe almost all emphasize the development of personality in the first-year course. Presumably one might consider other starting points, but keeping the time limitations in mind, I think that after a general introduction the subject of personality and its development is a logical place to begin. Along with this, the structural concept and the mental mechanisms are frequently introduced.

Next, and generally in the second year, psychopathology is taught. This is closely connected with the preceding year's work and leads to the work of the third and fourth years. In these latter two years the emphasis is on working with patients, but again a constant effort is maintained to integrate the material covered in previous years with current material.

Now to consider some of the possible methods of presenting the material. It would appear logical that if a teacher who knows his subject is also a gifted lecturer, there is no question but that he should lecture. Other methods include demonstrations of live human material, motion pictures, assigned reading, and group discussions.

In our experience the first-year course has been the subject of most discussion. Our staff considers it the most difficult to teach, and because it is the introductory course it is thought to be of special importance in that the attitude toward psychiatry which the student develops at this time may well be decisive for the rest of his career. The task of attempting to help medical students learn to recognize infantile sexuality, the unconscious, primary and secondary processes, repression, regression, conflict and defense, transference and countertransference is not an easy one. It is in the first-year course that the attempt is begun. I wish to emphasize what I have already stated—that it is the repeated presentation of the basic concepts in all four years that is apt to produce the highest degree of success. It is especially important that the underlying basic dynamics be demonstrated in patients.

The description of a first-year course as I shall present it is a bare outline and is intended to be viewed as a basis for discussion. After an introduction the subject of personality is considered. Following a discussion of the definition of personality, brief statements concerning the factors affecting personality up to the point immediately following birth are made. After that the theme of psychosexual development is traced, including the outlines of libidinal development, the formation of object relations, and ego development. At appropriate intervals demonstrations are presented, starting with a demonstration of two infants, each three or four days old, to show some of the differences which occur at this early age (e.g., differences in motility). Other demonstrations include mother-infant relationships, sibling relationships, children in the latency period, adolescents, etc.

From time to time carefully selected patients may be used in demonstrations to point up the relationship between certain symptoms and factors of development. For example, young patients with psychogenic megacolon are brought in with their mothers; usually it is fairly easy to illustrate effectively tensions and hostilities between the parent and child which highlight the conflict as it centers around the question of control.

The most effective method of presenting such material ultimately depends on the particular skills of the teachers. It is my opinion that demonstrations are especially effective, and that it is particularly important for first-year medical students to see people. Although there are some excellent motion pictures available they do not have the same impact that a live person generally does. It is my belief that the use of the small-group discussion is one of the most effective ways to teach this material. In this kind of situation the student and teacher have an opportunity to become better acquainted, in addition to which the teacher can more accurately gauge the differences between the students while giving each student the maximum of individual attention.

The value of the small-group discussion is effective in each of the four years. In the second year, where the student is introduced to patients for the purpose of his learning psychopathology, such discussion may be of great help in preventing anxiety which might otherwise permanently interfere with his working with such patients. In the third and fourth years, in addition to the small-group meetings, there are situations in which the student should have time alone with the instructor. Just how much time can be expended in this way depends largely on the number of teachers available.

I have stressed the importance of repeatedly presenting the basic concepts to the student through the work of the four years. In the clinical years, in his work with patients, he will have the best opportunity to check the validity of those concepts. Along with this emphasis on the importance of work continuity throughout all four years I believe that one of the principal means of accomplishing this is by making certain that there is a close, ongoing, working relationship between the members of the whole teaching team.

One of the most effective settings in which to teach dynamic psychiatry is in the outpatient clinic where arrangements are made for the student to follow at least one or two patients for as long as one school year. Such a situation, where the student can study the patient intensively and at the same time receive adequate supervision, is conducive to the testing out and confirmation of many basic concepts. Here it is possible for him to observe the unconscious fantasies and the related patterns of behavior. He has an opportunity to see the expression of affects and the defenses against them. In short, the outpatient clinic provides him with objective evidence that the experiences of infancy and early childhood do in fact affect the behavior of adult life.

Along with the experience in the adult outpatient clinic, it is important that the medical student be given the opportunity to work with children. If at all possible, this should include infants seen in well-baby clinics and young children seen in nursery and elementary school, as well as sick children in the outpatient clinic and hospital. Here too the medical student is in a position to see the raw data from which the theoretical concepts are derived.

In addition to work done in the department of psychiatry, it is sometimes possible to help the student learn from his work with patients in other departments. This may be accomplished directly by having psychiatric instructors or consultants available on other services, or indirectly by encouraging the student to describe his patients on the other services. Obviously, the extent to which this goal is achieved is in large part dependent on the cooperation of other members of the faculty.

The area of psychosomatic illness is of particular importance. It is important as a setting for the student to learn something about the relationship between emotional elements or forces and somatic responses. It is precisely in this area, however, that the student is likely to form erroneous conceptions which, instead of deepening his knowledge, do just the opposite. There have been strong tendencies to oversimplification in connection with psychosomatic conditions which tend to give the student a false sense of security. It is here also that the emphasis may be shifted away from dynamic psychiatry to a rigid set of "rules of thumb," which can mislead the student and interfere with his understanding of the dynamic process.

One subject which needs to be considered in connection with the discussion of teaching and learning dynamic psychiatry is that of reading material. Should a textbook be used? If not, what should be suggested or required? Here again I believe that the final decision should be made only after taking several factors into account, for example, the amount of faculty time available and the amount of attention which can be given to individual students. From a practical point of view, the selection of the best text available together with a list of selected readings seems to be a partial solution. In addition, given a situation in which the teacher knows the student well enough, other books and papers may be recommended specifically for individual students.

In connection with reading, there is another large source of valuable information—the world of literature. Although most medical students seldom have the time for anything other than technical reading, it is possible for the teacher of dynamic psychiatry to draw upon literary content with which the student has had previous acquaintance, or to suggest some work which might be read when the student does have time. Such reading may include novels, poetry, or plays. In essence, I am recommending that the student be referred to the work of the artist in the attempt to further his understanding of human behavior. Using this material, it seems to me, encourages medical students to maintain a broad and open attitude while helping them to see the relationship of these humanistic works to the most humane of all studies—the study of medicine.

SUMMARY

With the discovery and development of psychoanalytic concepts there has evolved an important area of the application of these concepts in the field of medicine generally and in the field of psychiatry particularly. These ideas have not always been received warmly, but during the past 20 years the opportunities for psychoanalytically trained people to teach in medical schools have increased greatly.

The experience of the past 20 years indicates that this teaching has probably been carried out with varying degrees of success. It is now the task of the teacher to examine this experience with the hope that it may be improved upon in the future. I have expressed some ideas and opinions regarding the teacher, the student, and the milieu in which they work together with some suggestions that I hope will prove helpful.

Discussion

DR. BANDLER: Dr. Tidd devotes two-thirds of his comprehensive paper to significant general issues relevant to medical education, the milieu, the goals and philosophy of medical education, and the nature of the student and faculty. He devotes one-third to the specific questions of the teaching of dynamic psychiatry, to the psychiatric curriculum, and to methods of teaching. I thoroughly agree with Dr. Tidd's emphasis and would conclude that these general issues of medical education are the crucial factors in determining the success of teaching dynamic psychiatry to the majority of medical students. Dr. Tidd defines our goals as providing "the medical student with information which will enable him to understand as well as possible the mental and emotional elements of human personality and human illness."

This is no modest goal that we set ourselves. It includes the assimilation of this information, the student's capacity to integrate it in his daily functioning as a physician, the development of attitudes, the growth of ego, the recognition of feelings both in others and himself, and the development of a

Drs. Bernard Bandler, Douglas D. Bond, and Alfred H. Stanton delivered prepared discussions by invitation.

Drs. Lawrence S. Kubie, Milton Rosenbaum, Albert J. Solnit, Charles W. Tidd, Thomas F. Dwyer, Frank Haendel, Theodore Jacobs, Arthur F. Valenstein, and Gregory Rochlin took part in the general discussion.

more comprehensive identity as a physician than is otherwise expected by many of the other disciplines of the medical school. With the exception of those students who plan to continue in psychiatry, I suspect that we are not too successful in achieving our goal. For evidence I will simply cite the experience of most psychiatrists throughout the country who are involved in the training of nonpsychiatric interns and residents; that is, graduates of a medical school with a good teaching program in dynamic psychiatry. The first success of these programs mentioned is that the nonpsychiatric physician becomes less hostile to psychiatry and more compassionate and humane toward his patient.

On another occasion I have attempted to explain this phenomenon by referring to the lack of time available for educational working-through at the medical school, analogous in its way to the working-through in analysis. It was my impression that the student's knowledge of psychiatry was greater than manifested but had become latent. There are, however, I believe, other reasons for this phenomenon, and they are related to the broad issues which Dr. Tidd mentions: the goals and philosophy of medical education, the nature of the medical student, his evolving personality and his development of a professional identity in the milieu of the medical school.

By milieu at the medical school, Dr. Tidd refers principally "to the members of the faculty and their attitudes toward psychiatry." I would expand this concept of milieu somewhat to include: the total attitudes of administration and faculty toward medical education. These attitudes make up the educational climate which facilitates the learning process as well as personal and professional growth.

The milieu is very much affected by the goals and philosophy of medical education. Dr. Tidd in considering the goals in teaching dynamic psychiatry starts "with the question of the over-all goal of the medical curriculum." He answers this by saying that "the goal is to give the student as good a start as possible on the road to becoming a good physician." Some schools have as a major goal the production of teachers and research scientists. Others, while in agreement on the goal of a physician, disagree about the road to be followed. Some argue that the goal at medical school is to educate students in respect to scientific principles. The patient, his family and his milieu, the doctor-patient relationship, home medical services, using ambulatory patients for teaching, and psychiatry are often looked upon as secondary by exponents of this point of view. Such thing, they say, belong not to the science of medicine but to the art which would be acquired in the course of internship and residency.

The goals and philosophy of a school are also reflected in the sequence and content of the student's educational experiences throughout the four years. I believe that this is crucial in the first two years. The nature of the experiences and the types and varieties of the models who are his teachers play significant roles in channeling the student's personal growth and early professional identification.

One sequence which tends to place exclusive emphasis on the traditional basic sciences in the first year and a half offers the student implicit values and attitudes as well as a characterization of the nature of a physician. The teachers are largely basic scientists. The orientation tends to be chiefly biological, not psychobiological, organic rather than functional, and reductionist in respect to understanding biological processes rather than multidetermined; that is, it recognizes the psychological and social dimensions as well as the

[58]

biological. The basic scientists and the cadaver, whose place in medical education and in the identity of the physician has been written about so brilliantly by Dr. Bertram Lewin, are often the major models placed before the student.

The psychology of the personality in such a curriculum is not usually considered a basic science. Although psychiatry is included in the first year, it is more often regarded as a clinical science. This attitude, which is independent in many ways of the degree of friendliness to psychiatry manifested by any individual faculty member, is reinforced for the student by the modest curricular time allocated to it. The student knows which are the important subjects he has to pass if he is to succeed in his very elemental struggle for survival at medical school. He knows which ones demand the greatest concentration and which ones can be glossed over in terms of his time budget. He knows that no one has been flunked out of medical school in the first two years because of his failure in psychiatry.

Dr. Tidd discusses at some length the nature of first-year medical students, emphasizing their ability to approach the study of medicine with eagerness, enthusiasm, freshness, and vigor. I agree that this may be the way they are on the first day at medical school. But how long does it last? What happens thereafter? To what extent is the student's maturation and development of an identity as a physician affected in its specificity by the milieu, by the goals and philosophy of the curriculum, by the permanence of anatomy and the cadaver in the first year, by the fact that the major models in the first two years are often basic scientists, and by the work overload? I should like to emphasize the work overload as possibly the single most decisive and crucial factor in the personal development of the student, his growing identity as a physician and, as a result, in the teaching of dynamic psychiatry to medical students. There is

[59]

considerable evidence indicating that the initial freshness, enthusiasm, earnestness, and vigor demonstrated by the medical student is of short duration; at some medical schools these qualities last from September in the first year to November, a total of about eight weeks.

What is the evidence? *Boys in White* (Becker *et al.*, 1961) is a book about student culture in medical school written by four eminent social scientists after five years of intensive study of a state school in Kansas. They describe three perspectives developed by the first-year student in the course of his first eight weeks at school—the initial, the provisional, and the final. The initial perspective is enthusiastic and educationally idealistic: learning is everything; it is recognized that there is a tremendous amount to be learned; there is determination to work very hard and, if that is not enough, to somehow work harder.

The provisional perspective is marked by the recognition that not everything can be learned in the time available, and that selection is necessary according to two criteria of importance: either by that which is fantasied to be important in medical practice, or that which the student thinks that the faculty wants him to know. The student's goal of learning, of education, begins to weaken and the attitude toward faculty begins to shift from the original image as educational allies to an impersonal "They."

The final perspective establishes the criterion of importance as that which the faculty wants the students to know. This is the way of survival which will enable the student to pass examinations and to get through school. Everything short of cheating is fair in the effort to find out what questions will be asked on the examination. The student continues to work hard, but his zest and enthusiasm are gone. His educational goal has been replaced by the goal of memorizing, much to the despair of the faculty members who complain that the student is not interested in learning. The student becomes entrenched in his vision of the faculty as "They"—the opponents who are to be outwitted.

I could offer various reasons to support my contention that the book's conclusions are valid only for the particular school which was studied, and I could think of many students to whom its conclusions do not apply. Last year, however, at Boston University, a tutorial program was instituted at the medical school. This program was entrusted to the Division of Psychiatry for first-year medical students. Curriculum time of an hour and a half a week was assigned to the tutorial program, whose goals were over-all educational, and not the teaching of psychiatry. We had seven tutors, each with a group of 10 to 11 students. To our amazement, *Boys in White* came alive under our eyes. We were able to observe the effects of the work overload on the development of attitudes, on the hardening of the defenses of the ego, on the need to control and repudiate feelings rather than recognize them, and on the beginning identity of a physician, effects that were antithetic to the goals of teaching dynamic psychiatry to medical students. I should add that it was also our impression that the tutorial experience was to some extent a partial educational corrective of the overload problem.

I hope that Dr. Tidd's emphasis on general educational issues will lead us to devote more time to their study. There is no danger of our neglecting the study of the psychiatric curriculum and our teaching methods, the student and his psychiatric teacher. But, just as in our therapy we are ascribing increasing importance to the family, and in our ward treatments to the milieu, so in the teaching of dynamic psychia-

[61]

try I believe we should devote more study and thought to the goals and philosophy of the curriculum, to the milieu of the medical school, to the specifics of the maturation of the medical student, and to the processes by which he arrives at his professional identity.

The teaching of dynamic psychiatry has important implications with respect to the nature of the physician and to the growth of the student in relation to the educational process. If there is harmony between the educational process in the medical school and the educational process in the psychiatric curriculum, then I believe it is possible to teach dynamic psychiatry successfully to the majority of students. If these processes, however, are not synchronous, if there are clashes, tensions, and contradictions between the goals and philosophy of medical education and those of psychiatric education, if the milieu of the medical school offers one ideal and the milieu of psychiatry offers another, then the student is caught in an educational conflict. I think there is little doubt as to how that conflict will be resolved by the majority of students or how seriously it will jeopardize their learning of dynamic psychiatry. Such conflicts, as we know, are not inevitable. And we can contribute to their solution by devoting more of our efforts to the basic problems of medical education.

DR. BOND: I do not suffer from the same complaint that others do. I think there are several things that my position as a Dean has brought to light, things that I wouldn't have known otherwise.

Throughout much of our thinking we sound as if we had a terrible envy of the basic scientist; we sound as if the basic scientist were winning the day—as if he set the model for medical students to follow, as if he lived in the field of certainty, while we live in the field of uncertainty. This is simply an illusion. There is an enormous resistance on the part of the medical student to learning any basic science whatsoever. He says: "What good is this nonsense? How can I use it? How can I use the Krebs cycle to treat a patient?" The basic scientists suffer from the resistance that students show toward them. They feel that the clinical people hold sway, and there is not much doubt that the clinical people do. Furthermore, how many medical students go into basic science? Not more than three to five per cent, and of that three to five per cent there is *probably* one per cent that is really good. How many people go into psychiatry from medical school? Hundreds. The psychiatrist has had a field day at recruiting people for his field, but I am not sure that we recruit all the people we should and could.

One of the troubles with the papers we have to discuss is that they are hard to fight with. I think that they are thoughtful, and that they are comprehensive. On the other hand, I think that some of them miss some points.

Psychoanalysis holds a peculiar position, and in many ways we psychoanalysts are a combination of many things. We feel that we have a basic science, and we feel we also have a clinical application. We have a difficult time because we are interested in the body of knowledge and theory that analysis has collected—and we are particularly strong on the theory. At the same time, we are a clinical field that tries to be therapeutic, with more or less success. We are caught in a position similar to that of a physiologist, if, while he studies the workings of the human body, he inadvertently creates a therapeutic effect. In a way, it is a shame that we are not more separate. If we could have an honest basic-science field in which we studied the mechanisms of the human mind and, as we clarified the issues, did not worry about application at all,

[63]

then we could take some of this knowledge and apply it to the treatment or to the management of the patient. But we have a combined field, and this gives us a certain amount of theoretical difficulty.

There are a few other things. When I first became a professor of psychiatry, I ran into Ernst Kris, who said, "Look, there are two things that you have to remember. There are only two ways, two features of the human mind, that you can use to overcome resistance; one is the intellect and the other is positive transference." If you insult the intellect and get a negative transference, it is not going to be a big surprise if people do not learn from you. I think that many people who start to teach think that it will be easy, particularly because they think they know what they want to say. Once they become actively involved, they are not so sure what it is they want to say, and usually they pay not the slightest attention to what the student wants to hear. This is rather important because, if the student doesn't want to hear it, he is not going to learn it. It is a little reminiscent of the Thurber story of a third-grade girl who was given a book on seals by her teacher and went off and read it. The teacher asked her if it was a good book. She said, "Yes, it is a good book." The teacher asked her if she liked the book. The child said, "No, I hated the book." "Why?" said the teacher. "Because it told me more about seals than I wanted to know."

I think it is characteristic of many consulting analysts that, if a surgeon calls and says, "Should I operate on this patient or shouldn't I operate on this patient?" they are likely to tell that surgeon a lot of stuff he doesn't want to know. Usually they forget to say, "Yes, operate on him," or "No." In regard to teaching, we are also much more likely to tell than to show. This is a big problem. We are interested in a lot of things

[64]

because they are shown to us by patients. But many of our patients drop down a big, deep well as far as the referring physician is concerned. Many of the things we are particularly interested in seeing, and perhaps in demonstrating, take place in secret. This is unfortunate from the teaching point of view.

I have a fine illustration of this sort of thing from Jack Flumerfelt. Caught between hours, he was persuaded by a house officer to see a patient who was delirious. Pressed for time, he flipped over the chart and noticed that the delirium was periodic. He also noticed that each delirium followed a rectal instillation made a few minutes earlier. He said one thing to the house officer: "Do you have to give that rectally? Don't!" With that, he was off.

The next day the house officer was banging on his door, exclaiming, "It's a miracle."

Jack said, "That's nice. That's what we're here for."

The house officer answered, "How did you know that did it?"

"I didn't know. It was just a shot in the dark."

"Not so, Doc," the house officer said.

"You know, some people don't like to have stuff stuck up . . . ."

"Is that right?" said the kid.

"That's right."

"What kind of people?" asked the kid.

"What kind of a fella is the guy we're talking about?"

The house officer replied, "A fellow sitting in an unrumpled bed, extremely neat, very neat little moustache, etc., with a little bit of femininity about him."

Jack said, "That's the kind. Remember it!"

The thing that is extremely nice is that if you can show them your effectiveness, then they are interested. You have to arouse

[65]

a certain amount of curiosity or show a certain amount of success before anybody is interested. For instance, I've often thought: What if we were running a psychiatric ward about 1937, with a number of pneumonia patients on it? Some over-eager fella whom we barely know comes over from the basic-science department and says, "I've got a lot of fungus juice here, and I'd like to stick it in one of your patients." We would say, "Fungus juice! These people are sick enough. Get out of here." If, on the other hand, he persuaded us to use it on one patient and that patient got well, we might get interested too.

I want to talk about one other matter. As you know, in our curriculum at Western Reserve we developed a program in which the medical student meets a pregnant woman, visits the home, and watches the development of the child. There were several reasons why we decided to do this. I'm not sure you know one of the most important reasons. We thought it important to understand the student, what he finds traumatic, and why he closes his eyes as he goes through the curriculum. We are interested in dynamic causes, and I thought that after my experience with young fliers in the war there might be considerable trauma connected with the cadaver. After all, we are taught for 20 years to respect our own body and the bodies of others. And suddenly a student comes to medical school, is presented with a body, and told to dissect it. Our predecessors had the advantage of kneeling down at the head of the departed and praying to God for forgiveness for what they were about to do. (You can be sure that added to the prayer there was a little rider that said: "I hope my body doesn't end up here too.") This was a regular ritual. We are not so blessed with this ritual and don't practice it. It is striking how medical students deal with this trauma. They are likely to shut right down in their thinking; they are likely to shut right down in the way they approach the cadaver. In the beginning they become extremely interested in one square millimeter of skin, and for a very good reason. They do not want to think of themselves as hurting a human body. Later, they are apt to respond with bravado—very much the way young fighter pilots respond with bravado to the death that surrounds them—and retreat into a regressive vulgarity: "Why go out to lunch? Here's a piece of liver." Or they may remove various parts of the cadaver and send it as a present to a friend. It is clear why they do this: they are coping with their reaction to death. This is one of the reasons we thought it wise to start with a pregnant woman: we start with life, not death. Psychologically, we feel this is a much sounder approach. We also think (although I do not know how one proves this with so many other things going on at the same time) that this approach has resulted in a much greater openness on the part of the student.

For instance, I remember clearly my own reaction when as a college student I went to see Harvey Cushing operate. It was a very frightening experience. A man with his head shaved, lying face down, was wheeled into the theater. He looked a little like a pig. His wife and child were sitting in the anteroom. Everything was all right until the first cut was made. At this moment, one remembers the wife, the child, and the patient and thinks: "My gosh, what's this man going to go through? The human tragedy of the whole thing!" Then they crack the skull (which is very impressive because it does in fact crack), and I didn't know whether I was going to make it or not. Then a very nice thing happens; the drapes are arranged; the patient is covered; the hole is there—but now it is only a hole. And pretty soon you are thinking "Why don't they make that hole bigger so you can see better?" I think at this moment you lose your feelings, and your curiosity and interest are ex-

[67]

cited. However you lose some of the human element (you have to, perhaps) before you're ready to inquire.

DR. STANTON: The comments on both Dr. Tidd's and Dr. Dwyer's papers about psychoanalysis as a science seem to me to represent the advantage of teaching in the medical school or in an academic setting. As anybody who has done teaching knows, this setting does not lend itself to an unquestioning, routine imparting of information. Questions are raised by various able questioners, including yourselves, and it is these questions which feed back into psychoanalysis and psychiatry with considerable potential gain.

To speak of just one aspect of what the preceding papers have discussed: medical faculties and medical schools are much concerned with the question of "basic science." The first word in that phrase, "basic," suggests a host of troubles. The first and most important cause of trouble is that it is a sort of icon and at the same time it has no clear meaning. That is, the word "basic" is used very often, most importantly perhaps to bring about an effect, wittingly or unwittingly. One reinforces a prejudice under the guise of giving information. When occasionally one hears the term coupled with an equally empty emotional term—"basic fundamentals"— usually mentioned in a lower voice, one is tempted to go into some full ritual. I mention this to suggest that in contrast it is possible to consider science as science; perhaps good or bad, exact or inexact, of known practical use or none—but these are other and clearer conceptions than "basic" science.

A second meaning is found in the medical-school schedule. A "basic science" is conceived of as a more fundamental one in the hierarchy of sciences from chemistry and physics up to biology, psychology, and the like. This meaning is by no means

[68]

empty, but it does incidentally imply a substantial body of knowledge which permits psychological phenomena to be predicted from biological. In addition to such information, there are indications that certain aspects of subjective experience— the social and the cultural—will never be reducible in any simple sense to the biology of the individual. It is this point that the psychiatrist advances as ground for conceiving the historical, ecological, and social sciences as basic also to the psychologic.

A third meaning is not immediately pertinent to Dr. Dwyer's topic. "Basic" may imply the empirical testing and the grounds for theory. Psychoanalytic theory, for instance, ranges from the clinical to the almost philosophical, as noted by Waelder. Many expect that the next significant developments in psychoanalysis are apt to come from testing in application, and even from the development of the appropriate measurements and objective statistical analyses which have been met with so much suspicion by clinical theorists. This is more likely to develop from the testing of the clinical theory than it is from the more metapsychological variables. Systematic empirical analysis is the wellspring of new findings and new theories, not merely testing grounds for familiar theories. The case, with relatively long-term contact between a supervised student and one patient, remains a most pertinent and effective means for enabling the student to grasp our methods. I say this because I am going to turn my attention to first-year teaching, where case observation is likely to be mixed intimately with treatment and with the clinic.

The other methods of empirical analysis applicable to psychiatric and psychoanalytic theory will draw heavily and profitably from methods useful in psychology and the social sciences as well as from the methods of the biological sciences.

[69]

These sciences are basic to psychoanalysis. It is to the detriment of both the sciences and psychoanalysis that physicians may complete their full undergraduate and medical work without any exposure whatsoever to these disciplines in premedical work and in the medical school. This constitutes a major threat insofar as psychological medicine will become a practitioner-dominated art, a school of psychological operators interested in refinements and techniques dictated by the clinical outcome, without the disciplined and practical knowledge of the procedures necessary to develop the science. Under such circumstances, it seems to me highly possible that major developments will come primarily from the other side of the river, with medical men serving as technicians. I do not, therefore, believe that one can include materials from the social and behavioral sciences at the expense of teaching psychoanalysis or psychiatry.

From this general consideration, a question arises regarding one of Dr. Dwyer's suggestions. Work in the first two years should focus on the phenomena of stress in relatively normal persons, phenomena that the student will recognize from his own experience. We will always deal with students who bring their past experience with them to the seminars, but to the extent that one relies on the personal experience of the student without adequate theoretical and empirical development, one risks the student's remaining trapped by the language and concepts of the folk psychology which he learned at his mother's knee. He will have learned, for instance, that many things (e.g., homosexuality) do not exist when in fact they do. Dr. Bibring once called attention to homosexual living as a major problem which was not touched upon anywhere in the medical curriculum in certain schools. I should like, therefore, to emphasize the need for supplementing any self-recognition with the tools of intellectual mastery: good systematic theory and empirical grounds stated in terms which have been defined not privately but according to the canons of scientific criticism (such as the list of definitions of the defenses which has come from the Beth Israel group). Such a learning procedure will not be entirely pleasant or even immediately understandable to all students, but experience would suggest that such training would provide tools for opening doors to the future development of the science. After all, a major criterion for the appraisal of a science or theory and of an educational system is the type of program which is written for the development and improvement of the science itself. It calls for a reasonable grounding in both the range of phenomena and the theory before attempting to confront the problems of the clinic.

I have focused very narrowly upon the issue of teaching theory and its relatively systematic application, primarily because it seems to me that in the presentations so far presented the important place of disciplined thought has not been sufficiently stressed. It has not, however, been my intention to question the relevancy of its applications to the really personal, to real human beings.

* * *

Dr. Kubie: Many generalizations are made about the processes of change in medical students, but except for the one interesting study (Becker *et al.*, 1961) mentioned by Dr. Bandler there have been no systematic studies of these processes. It is obvious that we need funds for basic research in this area. Such funds would enable us to conduct a study of a random, statistically adequate sample of medical students from different medical schools through the four years of their

[71]

medical education, and perhaps for several years afterwards. This kind of project is currently being considered by a number of engineering schools. The sampling factors that would be involved in such a study and the techniques to be used are obvious. But there are many important problems requiring clarification, such as the significance of the differences in dropout rates from different medical schools, and dropouts from these as a whole as compared with those from engineering and law schools. If we are going to relate our educational process to what goes on in other fields of graduate education, some such basic studies will have to be made.

It is as difficult for a school to study itself as it is for an individual to study himself. Indeed a school cannot study itself objectively. We therefore need an interschool agency to conduct such studies. Furthermore, it is essential that the material gathered in such a study must not get back to the schools themselves, because such a practice would seriously impair the investigators' chances of obtaining accurate information from most students, not to mention the faculties. This is another reason for an independent interschool agency.

One of the basic issues is the importance of self-knowledge. It is interesting to note that we do not use psychoanalytic training as our model in this connection. I do not mean to say that this model is necessarily the only one or the best one (perhaps it is not the best even for analysis); but certainly it is a model that ought to be considered in connection with the training of medical students. Nor should we keep silent about it merely because it is difficult to achieve. The late Bill Clark was a professor of surgical pathology at the College of Physicians and Surgeons of Columbia University in New York. When he was not practicing surgical pathology, he was a crusty old farmer, given to muttering that he would not let anybody into medical school who had not been analyzed. I do not think that most of us would go so far as to recommend that every applicant to medical school be analyzed. But if we believe that self-knowledge in depth is part of the affective maturational process, we should seek other means to achieve the same analytical objective.

One approach to this problem has been wholly overlooked. When it dropped out of existence, it also dropped out of everybody's thinking. This approach was used at Emory Medical College under Carl Whitaker, between 1944 and 1950. The department of psychiatry was young and irregular in its training, but it faced up to this problem with a greater courage and honesty than any of us has shown since then. The medical students were divided into small groups of about six students, each group led by one of the members of the psychiatric staff. Throughout the four years, they met every Saturday morning for sessions of group therapy. Although there is certainly something naïve about this approach, if any of you had had the opportunity to study it closely as I did, you would have found much that was impressive and little to scoff at. The fact that the sessions were eventually dropped is no reason for turning up our noses, or for turning away from the search for methods by which this aspect of the growth process can be brought into medical education.

Dr. Rosenbaum: I would like to talk about humanism. I think that we must start out fully aware of the fact that neither psychoanalysis nor psychoanalysts are particularly humanistic. If we are to discuss humanism in terms of those involved in certain social issues, then my guess is that medical faculties are, by and large, humanistic, and so are analysts on those medical faculties, but that practicing analysts or analytic in-

[73]

stitute faculties are not necessarily so. That is not a criticism, but somehow we have an idea that we analysts are more concerned about people than any of our colleagues, and it simply is not true. In teaching, we have to do away with these moral value judgments which imply that somehow we are more humanistic, somehow better people. When you ask the question (Dr. Bandler brought this out beautifully), "How do you get the students involved?" it is my feeling that we have already gone through the "popularity contest" phase of our development. It was not easy for us when we first started to teach in medical schools. So, the first thing we had to do was make ourselves liked. The easiest way to do that was to throw patients at the students in the first year—even the pregnant women. Perhaps we are mature enough, now that we have a body of content. But we still have no textbook. The department of biochemistry has a textbook; the department of physiology has, and so have the others. It is rather interesting that we do not.

Consider the milieu of the student. What did the boys who came to us from top-notch schools do in their junior and senior years? They were working in small seminar groups. But medical school is like high school, and boys who come to us from a city college are apt to make a better adaptation in the beginning. Therefore, I think that we in psychiatry ought to use some high-school methods, too.

I should like to consider one other thing: the student's commitment to medicine. If you commit yourself to being a doctor, then there are certain things you have to do. If I introduce certain basic psychological principles like that of self-knowledge, I introduce it not because I want to make the student a better person (maybe it will), but because self-knowledge is as important in his work with patients as is knowing some-

[74]

thing about biochemistry. After introducing the content, you can bring in any number of experiments in the laboratory to show what happens to the blood pressure of a patient when the doctor leaves or when he gets mad. Thus psychological principles are presented in much the same way, let us say, as are those of biochemistry. The teacher of biochemistry will say: "This is important; this is a body of content." Douglas D. Bond is perfectly right. The students dislike the basic sciences—and we know what happens to those students. Even in those schools in which the faculty is so concerned about the image of basic sciences, not all students have the same goal, not all have the same image of themselves in the future.

I should like to make a final point, one that has not been given proper emphasis: students should be informed that analysts differ from one another, and that these differences are relevant. A psychoanalyst who is affiliated with an institute and who is a practitioner is not the same as a psychoanalyst who has a full-time position in the medical school. He cannot be the same. He has to change. The psychoanalyst in the department of psychiatry has become interested in social psychiatry and in teaching analysis. Perhaps the role of a biochemist is pretty much the same, inside or out of the medical school. But I think that teaching analysis in the medical school requires a type of person who is basically different from the outside analyst.

DR. SOLNIT: I would like to point to yet another emphasis inferred from Dr. Tidd's and Dr. Dwyer's papers: the struggle between what might be called the molecular view and what might be called the macroscopic view, whether in biology or chemistry, clinical medicine or surgery, or in psychiatry. As Dr. Stanton implies, I think we have to drop the term "basic," because it obscures rather than clarifies our consideration of what is going on. In biology, there is just as heated a controversy under way right now between the naturalists and the molecular biologists as there is in our own field. Our controversy centers on the question: are we going to emphasize applications and the way in which these applications sharpen our vision, or are we going to emphasize "microscopic" studies in depth? It seems to me a healthy controversy. Moreover, we must be aware of this controversy, if we are going to face the problems of curriculum. I think Dr. Bond's cutting edge both helps us and obscures from us a realization that it is impossible at present, in a four-year curriculum, to produce an all-American physician complete, with the scientific, physical, psychological, and social aspects of medical knowledge, and equipped for medical care. Dr. Kubie has given considerable thought to this problem and has written about it from one point of view. I think that we have to look at it not only in terms of psychiatry, but also in terms of training the internist, the pediatrician, and the surgeon. I suspect that the critical question should include not only "What should we teach?" but "What shouldn't we teach?"

DR. TIDD: I would like to re-emphasize that our staff has been most concerned with the first-year course in psychiatry, with what to teach and how to teach it. We are trying to introduce material from the behavioral sciences, but time limitations make this difficult. We are faced with the same sort of problem our colleagues in other departments are working on, for example, how to deal with the great amount of information in the field of molecular biology.

It seems to me that we would be doing a real service if we could convince our colleagues in other disciplines that material from the behavioral sciences would help to make better doctors in general and that such material is basic to the whole field of medicine, not just to psychiatry. Perhaps in that way we get more time in the curriculum either in premedical education or in the first and second years of medical school.

As to Dr. Bandler's remarks about work overload for the students, I suspect that most medical faculties are trying to do something about this—I know that we are. As a matter of fact, we are trying to clear up scheduled time to the point that there may be a little time left over for thinking and contemplating.

DR. DWYER: I agree with most of Dr. Bandler's remarks, although I would prefer to think that the students can retain their capacity for enthusiastic learning even under the overload of courses in the first two years, and even under the onslaught of hostile faculty members. I have had the opportunity to see fourth-year students retain this kind of optimism in spite of such influences, but the study in Kansas was of course more carefully systematic.

Dr. Bond has called attention to the difficulties that are created for psychoanalytic teachers and research workers because they are usually required to come forward with the goods—the clinical proof. This is an attitude not generally conducive to sound research. Unfortunately I have no solution to the problem. Ideally, there ought to be psychoanalysts (and this is a contradiction in terms) who are not doing psychoanalysis but who are doing research in psychoanalytic problems. I do not know what kind of people these would be, but there ought to be analysts who are not forced to come to a conclusion prematurely—prematurely from the point of view of research, not from the point of view of treatment. Dr.

Solnit has pointed to the fact that the struggle is heated among the biologists, too—the struggle over whether biology will be presented to the students as macroscopic or molecular. I think we can learn from some of their discussions.

DR. HAENDEL: I am a second-year resident for the Massachusetts General-McLean Hospital resident program. I want to comment on something Dr. Tidd mentioned. The matter of student resistance to learning dynamic concepts is clearly an important issue, as the very foundation of psychiatric practice rests on these theories. It seems to me that one of the major reasons for resistance is due to the approach brought to teaching by the psychiatrists. I refer to the frequent implication that certain concepts are regarded as substantive rather than as models. To illustrate: the structural hypothesis concerned with "defining" the id, ego, and superego is often misunderstood as having material location somewhere or other. In moments of reflection, we recognize that the id, just as the "mind," implies processes rather than places. To the medical student who is used to connecting concepts with laboratory proof of physical existence, this model may encounter the resistance of disbelief. Perhaps if our teachers of psychiatry were more explicit about the use of models as models, the student's resistance would be diminished.

DR. JACOBS: I should like to make two points. Dr. Dwyer has mentioned the importance of presenting psychoanalytic concepts to medical residents and other house officers in a meaningful way. He has spoken of the difficulty of presenting material directly from the couch. We all know that this is true, but it is no less true for teaching in the first two years of medical school. Material that may be highly sophisticated in psychoanalytic terms, but which is presented in a meaningless or complicated way to the student, often falls flat. So we have to think in terms of motivating the students to accept this material. We have found that the judicious use of material on patients is extremely helpful in this regard. After all, patients really constitute the laboratory for psychological courses in the first two years of medical school. We have found, as Dr. Rosenbaum mentioned, that simply introducing patients in order to become more popular with the students has not been effective at all. But to use patients, either from the emergency room or the wards, to illustrate the material we are trying to teach *is* important and helpful to the students. Not only are patient demonstrations useful, but allowing students to interview and talk to patients themselves is particularly important.

I have noticed that in this panel there has been little discussion of the problems associated with the third and fourth years of medical school. Perhaps this is because the problems are less acute, or because we have mastered some of the problems of those years. But there are some problems that I consider to be important in the clinical years. We have found that students who are faced with the hostile patient, or with the dying patient, or with the seductive patient, will often turn away from such patients, and avoid any contact with them. I find that this kind of medical patient offers a particularly effective means for teaching dynamic psychiatry. In our program, a psychiatrist meets with a small group of students throughout the entire junior year, and we have found that the positive relationship between instructor and student which evolves during a year's continuing association between the two has helped the student to master his anxieties about his patients and to develop in himself the psychological sensitivity that should be cultivated in all physicians.

DR. VALENSTEIN: Dr. Tidd has remarked that teaching and learning are certainly not the same, and, as a conceptual matter, I think it important to differentiate the two. They are complementary, and ideally they should be exactly reciprocal. Of course, they never are, but the degree of reciprocity depends to a large extent upon the sensitivity, skill, and versatility of the teacher, for he has the greater control of the situation.

The student should not be expected to set the stage, for it is primarily up to the teacher to understand the setting in which he presents his propositions, and to take into account not only the predilections and biases of the student, but also the administrative considerations influencing the curriculum, as well as the issues particular to the historical moment of his subject. The oscillations of history affect our cause with respect to what we teach, but our confidence that what we feel has scientific validity should not be shaken, even though the analytic point of view might go out of fashion to some extent. Entirely too much was expected of analysis in the first place. In that respect, it is a blessing that analysis as a therapeutic panacea is no longer the fashion in psychiatry or the behavioral sciences. But our disillusionment with the overexpectations of the postwar period has led to an inappropriate devaluation of the analytic point of view.

It is important to discriminate, as Dr. Bond has pointed out, between psychoanalysis as a valid body of facts and theories, and psychoanalysis as a psychotherapy—both in the classical application of analysis, and in its application to the various dynamic psychotherapies. Beyond all else, it offers a unique perspective for an understanding of human development and behavior which is still valid, and which will probably continue to be meaningful so long as man is a social animal whose adaptation is learned in considerable measure out of experience and educational processes. Molecular considerations are certainly germane, but in this respect I doubt that psychoanalysis will ever be totally overbalanced or superseded by the molecular approach. It is essential to be aware of the possibilities inherent in the different approaches to human behavior, and to appreciate the contributions and limitations of each one.

With all this in mind, the instructor is in the best position to consider what to present to the student, when it will be best presented, and what are its propitious possibilities. I was struck especially by Dr. Bond's emphasis (as well as Dr. Tidd's) on the first year. For that matter, the first part of the first year is especially crucial because the student has not yet formed self-protective attitudes which enable him to cope with disturbing experiences like "tearing apart" the previously sacrosanct human body. A relatively free access to the human body is habitually withheld, except under very special social sanction. The doctor is especially privileged with respect to the physical and emotional privacy of his patients, so long as he is professional in his approach, detached, objective, scientific, and above all, uninvolved emotionally, or at least not explicitly so.

There is, however, that brief period at the beginning of his medical training, when the student is in the first flush of enthusiasm, before he has adjusted his professional position to the intricacies of the human body and human behavior. What is presented during these early months has an important effect on the point of view he develops. The curriculum is decided by the department and by the medical-school administration, and the administration is susceptible to the spirit of the times, to what seems currently favorable, as they see it, for scientific research and development. Here comes the term "basic" again. Basic, molecular, impersonally scientific—all these considerations are relevant; nonetheless they should not supersede our own valid psychoanalytic position and perspective.

It comes down to the fact that in teaching one is limited by two sets of problems: those created by the learning potentialities of the student, and those associated with the teaching-learning atmosphere as influenced by the administration. The relationship between the two sets of problems is an intricate one, and becomes even more complex once the professionalization of the physician is well under way. By that time the medical student is deeply committed to patterning his attitudes and his professional position after the images set before him in the persons of his professors and instructors who may be overrepresented in his eyes as ideal.

DR. ROCHLIN: My teaching is confined to the later years of medical school. I have not had much direct experience with first- and second-year students. I would like to ask the speakers, as well as members of the panel, to what extent they institute or try to institute bedside teaching with the first- or second-year student (or even the third-year student) as coincident with making a physical diagnosis. Perhaps this is a well-explored and naïve question. However, I recall, for example, teaching clinical psychiatry on a medical ward—this opportunity is easily available, and is in no sense remote from the student's experience—to a group of second-year students at the bedside of a patient recovering from a coronary. Other disabilities common in the emergency room or the wards of any hospital provide excellent opportunities for teaching clinical psychiatry. To what extent have they been used?

I bring this up because many speakers have pointed to the difficulty of persuading medical students as to the validity of material that we know exists. I wonder if this difficulty may be partially related to the fact that the medical student is thrown directly into psychopathological material, or what he thinks is pathological, without the advantage of a workable frame of reference. It is too far removed as yet from his every-day experience. On the other hand, the experience of patients with hemiplegia, or injuries resulting from an accident, or patients in pregnancy, are very close to his immediate experience. These encounters require the student to travel only a short distance from his present orientation. In the hands of a competent analyst, this kind of material should not be difficult to demonstrate. I offer this as a question addressed to those concerned with the clinical part of the curriculum.

PANEL II: PSYCHIATRIC RESIDENTS

Chairman, HELEN H. TARTAKOFF, M.D.

D R. ROSENBAUM has mentioned that we have no textbook for the large subject of dynamic psychiatry. That is true. However, several books address themselves to this subject. A recent one, *Psychiatry and Medical Practice in a General Hospital* (Zinberg, 1964), has grown out of the combined experience of the psychiatric staff of the Beth Israel Hospital. I would like to quote from Dr. Bibring's preface to that book.

The Beth Israel Hospital in Boston is only one among many others that strive earnestly for the integration of modern medicine and psychoanalytic psychiatry in an ef- fort toward a deeper understanding of the sick person and of his illness. Though this may seem like a relatively limited program whose explicit objective varies from place to place, *implicitly* it aims toward *bridging the gap* beween the *organic* and the *psychological* concomitants in man—an endeavor that deserves infinite determination, patience and effort. As the different institutions explore this territory, whose boundaries are not drawn clearly and whose pathways are not yet marked carefully, they *each* develop their individual approach and their specific program according to their own prevailing interest and to the general constellation surrounding their work [p. xi].

The psychiatric resident, unlike the medical student, has declared himself for the field of psychiatry. If his commitment is soundly motivated, a unique educational experience awaits him. Unlike other specialists, he will stimulate change in others through the controlled utilization of his own personality. An empathic response to others based on self-knowledge has long been recognized as a means to this end. But psychiatric training requires far more than understanding based on insight. The resident's task will be facilitated greatly by the acquisition of certain essential skills and by a relevant set of guiding principles.

Psychotherapy: Models of the Essential Skill

RALPH J. KAHANA, M.D.

IN THE PAST 40 YEARS, largely under the impact of psychoanalysis, dynamic psychotherapy has become the principal
and essential curative skill of the American psychiatrist and,
increasingly, a focus of his training. As experience and information have accumulated, with a deepening and broadening
of psychoanalytic theory, the uses of psychotherapy have been
extended and refined. This well-founded growth has been
gradual and is, perhaps, in danger of being taken for granted.
It has influenced and responded to other developments in the
biological, clinical, and social sciences, and in the organization and administration of medical and psychiatric care.
Consequently, the indvidual psychiatrist now tends to concentrate on the psychotherapy of patients with particular disorders, or in certain age groups or settings, or on the
employment of selective approaches and techniques. The applications of psychotherapy have come to embrace: treatment

of psychoses and borderline states, impulse disorders and psychoneuroses; medical psychotherapy of emotional reactions to physical illness and psychosomatic disorders; psychotherapy of disorders or maturational crises of children, adolescents, or aging persons; psychotherapy in particular settings like social agencies, schools, colleges, industry, military service, or penal institutions; approaches of psychotherapy with pharmacological or physical treatments, hypnosis or in groups. Psychiatrists now collaborate in these efforts with workers in an increasing number of allied professional fields that use psychotherapeutic methods, including other branches of medicine and public health, clinical psychology, social work, child therapy, nursing, psychiatric aides, occupational therapy, remedial teaching, and educational, vocational, and pastoral counseling.

We may distinguish in the various uses and forms of psychotherapy certain interdependent methods and aims, basic therapeutic principles, determining conditions of psychotherapeutic relationships, and various kinds of clinical roles. Along with models[1] of psychic functioning and structure, of psychological development and adaptation, of personality types, of the genesis and forms of psychopathology, of psychotherapeutic techniques and patterns, and of different integrated styles of practice as embodied by instructors, these constitute the basic paradigms that we offer to the psychiatric resident as he gradually develops his own approach to actual

---

[1] The term "model" refers to: theoretic projections of a system of psychic functioning; descriptions of analogies that help in visualizing clinical relationships and trends and technical methods and objectives; examples of general types and common patterns; or persons and attributes worthy of imitation. A model may serve to organize instruction or may be directly presented to the trainee.

[88]

or potential patients in hospitals or in the community. The advance of psychotherapy in the general development of dynamic psychiatry has made the residency years more and more an introduction and preparation for a variety of possible careers. Thus it has become essential that instruction in psychotherapy be broad yet efficient. This paper will be devoted to consideration of some models that may help to meet these requirements, but first, in order to maintain an essential perspective, a few words should be said about the training experience.

THE STRESS OF PSYCHIATRIC TRAINING

Even the beginning resident who has been so fortunate as to have had basic dynamic psychology and the rudiments of psychopathology integrated in his medical training, including the effort to preserve his native empathy, curiosity, discernment, and tact, may reel under the initial impact of psychiatric training. The main stress is a concentrated exposure to the emotionally disturbed behavior of patients, especially states of extreme anxiety, despondency, helpless appeal, bizarreness or withdrawal, and attitudes of aggressive demandingness, provocativeness, or seductiveness (GAP, 1955). Later, this personal trial takes the form of subtle, sustained attraction and accurate attacks during longer contact with more perceptive and skillfully defensive patients. A second source of pressure lies in the technical task of carefully observing each patient, of understanding and evaluating him with increasing psychological depth, or remembering or recording interviews, and of guiding his own reactions in accordance with therapeutic aims, while at the same time responding with spontaneity as he and his patient get to know each other.

Added to these tasks are burdensome schedules, responsi-

[89]

bility for the care of suicidal, assaultive, acutely decompensating or chronically disabled people, the necessity to adapt to a competitive peer group and to confront the injunctions and judgments of his supervisors, and the almost limitless body of knowledge to be gained. The resident's response to such pressures affects his future capability as a psychotherapist even more than it influences his potential as a diagnostician, an administrator, or for certain kinds of research or teaching. These strains may be ameliorated, and the resident's learning enhanced, by appropriate dosage and timing of clinical experience and responsibilities, by the support of his peer group and his supervisors, by institutional arrangements, procedures, traditions and morale, through personal psychotherapy or psychoanalysis, and by the cumulative assimilation of information and techniques, organized and vitalized by theory.

The training experience raises many interesting questions of method and approach germane to a discussion of the psychotherapist's education such as these: Is it best for the resident to begin his clinical experience with the very sickest patients? Should didactic and theoretical instruction be emphasized (or indeed offered) at the beginning of residencies? What is the place of personal psychoanalysis in psychiatric training? For the present these questions will be passed by in order to concentrate upon certain teaching models.

MODELS OF PSYCHOTHERAPEUTIC METHODS AND AIMS

A wide range and variety of psychotherapeutic methods has long been recognized. Levine (1942) distinguished: the psychotherapeutic aspects of organic medical examinations and treatments, of hospitalization, and of occupational and recreational therapies; environmental steps to reduce strains and increase the satisfaction of needs; measures of acceptance, reassurance, guidance, limit setting, ventilation, desensitization and reeducation; and more formal psychotherapies. With the widening application of both psychoanalysis and dynamic psychotherapy to the entire spectrum of psychological malfunctioning, requiring technical and theoretical modifications, it became necessary to distinguish seemingly overlapping indications and methods. There was not only understandable confusion in the broad field of the psychotherapies, but also psychoanalysis itself as a relatively well-defined therapeutic tool and research method appeared to be threatened with dilution and distortion in consequence of efforts to expedite treatment and training (Benjamin, 1947). It was apparent that the aim of effecting profound changes within the three structural institutions of the mind (id, superego, ego) and in their reciprocal relations, through activation and interpretation of the infantile neurosis in the transference (E. Bibring, 1937), pertaining most typically to psychoanalysis of the hysterias and obsessional neuroses (the classical "transference neuroses"), was not generally feasible in dynamic psychotherapy, and was undesirable with certain kinds of psychopathology.

Apart from the use of psychotherapy as a stopgap when an analyst, or time, or money was unavailable or when the patient was in poor physical health, dynamic psychotherapy appeared to be more efficient in many cases as definitive treatment, or as preparation or follow-up to psychoanalysis. This was seen when illnesses were slight or transitory, were anchored in secondary gains, or entangled in the psychopathology of parents or marital partners, were too severe, or were attended by insufficient capacity for communication, trust,

[91]

insight, and other elements essential to therapeutic alliance, by too rapid and unstable developmental flux, or by advanced age limiting any great change in personality or making it inadvisable.

The frequent necessity to counter, or to at least avoid facilitation of regression, led in dynamic psychotherapy to the tendency to maintain a mild positive transference in an atmosphere of a temporary and relatively limited relationship, and to the use of face-to-face interviews which while focusing upon adaptation to currently stressful realities avoided the stirring up of inner conflicts (Benjamin, 1947; Stone, 1951). Knight (1949, 1952) polarized the aims of the psychotherapies as being on the one hand predominantly supportive, serving the reestablishment of those adaptive techniques that had at one time functioned most effectively, while on the other as mainly exploratory, essaying to deal with pathogenic conflicts short of therapeutic psychoanalysis. Gill (1954) suggested that the development of types of psychotherapy intermediate between full psychoanalysis and brief active therapy was consistent with a view of the psyche in which the outcome of struggles between drives and defenses had become crystallized into relatively enduring and autonomous ego organizations operating with neutralized energies. Thus intensive psychotherapy might alter relationships within the ego. Further, he raised the possibility that, even though basic conflicts may not be solved, derivative conflicts having relative autonomy might be worked out.

MODELS OF PSYCHOTHERAPEUTIC PRINCIPLES

Edward Bibring (1954), in a study with Grete L. Bibring (1947), delineated basic principles and procedures considered applicable to all methods of dynamic psychotherapy. Different forms of psychotherapy were characterized by a selective employment of the principles of *suggestion, abreaction, manipulation, clarification,* and *interpretation,* and by modification of the procedures of *production* of psychological material, the *utilization* of the material by the therapist (mainly) or the patient, the *assimilation* by the patient of the results of such utilization, and *reorientation* and *readjustment.* The principles are employed (1) technically to promote the treatment process, or (2) with directly curative intention. In therapeutic psychoanalysis, in which the main instrument of treatment is the interpretation of unconscious instinctual derivatives and defenses, the other principles are applied technically, thereby helping to achieve therapeutic alliance, maintain an optimum transference, encourage the patient to face his painful feelings and prepare the way for deeper self-understanding. Dynamic psychotherapy, lacking the ensemble of conditions which make interpretation effective—free association and auxiliary measures (Macalpine, 1950)—relies upon manipulation and upon the clarification of preconscious or conscious mental processes and contents. Suggestion and abreaction are used technically rather than curatively in psychotherapy, except in certain methods and conditions like hypnotherapy and acute traumatic reactions.

Manipulation—designating the employment of the patient's existing emotional systems (without relying upon a primitive transference relationship as in suggestion)—can be used to neutralize obstacles to treatment (such as an attitude of resentment) or to mobilize cooperation (as when we persuade a phobic patient to face what he fears). The term "manipulation" is not used in the deprecatory sense of "man-

[93]

aging fraudulently." In fact, it refers to the antithesis—approaching the patient with tactful appreciation of his viewpoint, experiences, needs and adaptive methods. The Bibrings have described two kinds of therapeutic manipulation. One refers to the patient's new experience in treatment, either in meeting an authority, the therapist, whose behavior is different from that which the patient has learned to expect and to fear from similar figures in the past, or in discovering that he himself can accomplish constructive changes which he had not believed possible. The "corrective emotional experience" (Alexander and French, 1946) may exemplify this method.

Another variety of therapeutic manipulation which Grete L. Bibring designates *adaptive intervention* refers to the redirecting of emotional forces toward adjustive change. It has manifold applications and a special place in residency training. The effectiveness of this method depends upon the extent to which the patient's personality and the adaptive tasks facing him can be understood. The personality diagnosis defines a characteristic, sustained pattern and range of perceptual, affective, cognitive, and conative responses to stress. It summarizes the history and outcome of the development of the individual's initially rudimentary sexual and aggressive drives and potential adaptive capabilities. This evolution is shaped by predetermined maturation, by the impact of the external world requiring the development of communicative, vocational, and other skills, by the necessary establishment of inner defenses against the urgent pressure of deep instinctual strivings, by the acquisition of environmentally influenced values and standards of behavior, and finally by a series of crucial inner conflicts.

We offer the psychiatric resident psychoanalytic paradigms

of personality structures as an orientation and a starting point for individual diagnosis (Kahana and G. L. Bibring, 1964). If a patient's response to stress remains confined to intensification of long-standing traits or minor symptoms, it may be sufficient for purposes of therapeutic management to comprehend his manifest attitudes as a function of his personality. A familiar example is the deliberately cooperative, even-tempered and effective compulsive person who has changed under pressure to a procrastinating, obstinate and controlling individual. Adaptive intervention might consist in respecting his autonomy by carefully and systematically structuring with him his role in overcoming the problems at hand, in recognizing his high standards, etc. Such curative applications of adaptive intervention have gained in scope and effectiveness from the enrichment of our knowledge of adaptation.

Since Freud's introduction of ego psychology, the adaptive point of view in psychoanalytic theory has been increasingly defined (Hartmann, 1939b, 1958; Rapaport and Gill, 1959). The meeting ground of psychology and the social sciences has been explored (e.g., Erikson, 1950). Adaptation has been examined in such specially traumatic and revealing situations as maternal deprivation, perceptual isolation, war, and concentration camps. Most useful of all to the psychiatric resident are clinical studies of critical phases of life, including criteria for successful adaptation. We can refer to the host of contributions in the fields of childhood development, puberty and adolescence (especially A. Freud, 1946, 1958; Erikson, 1950, 1959b), female psychology (H. Deutsch, 1944-1945), pregnancy (G. L. Bibring, 1959, and G. L. Bibring *et al.*, 1961), and aging. When personality structures are relatively unformed or unstable, as we find during childhood and in psychobiological life crises, then our therapeutic approach

rests more upon an appreciation of the particular maturational processes and adaptive challenges inherent in these
phases of existence.

Clarification helps the patient to recognize more accurately
his perceptions, feelings, and thoughts which he senses only
vaguely or hardly at all, to apprehend his symptoms and the
nature of his disorder, to appreciate causal and logical relationships, and to understand both his own attitudes and characteristic behavior patterns (now and as they have developed) as well as the personalities of the important people in
his life. When correctly applied, a clarification captures the
patient's interest and leads him to greater objectivity rather
than provoking defensiveness.

The ability to comprehend these preconscious elements
and to convey them to the patient is an essential psychotherapeutic skill to be developed in clinical training. This means
being familiar with the garden variety of daydreams and the
ordinary everyday human themes of love, competition, tri-
umph, failure, revenge, struggles of good versus bad, and the
like. In the realm of psychopathology, to take a well-known
example, the content of a depression may include: sensations
of fatigue, tension, anorexia and insomnia; feelings and
ideas of sadness, loss, helplessness, inadequacy, failure to meet
standards, self-hatred or barely concealed conceit, oversensi-
tivity, envy and spite, in addition to actions to compensate for
deprivation, to atone for guilt, or to avoid self-preoccupation
and self-pity. Depending upon the patient's personality structure and the therapeutic goals, it is frequently valuable to give
insight into such conscious or preconscious components,
whereas the more profound substratum of murderous rage
and introjection of lost objects may not become directly
interpretable.

[96]

MODELS OF THE PSYCHOTHERAPEUTIC RELATIONSHIP

Paralleling attempts to specify psychotherapeutic aims and methods are endeavors toward understanding the medium through which therapeutic principles are applied—the psychotherapeutic relationship in its various forms. Major determinants of psychotherapeutic relationships pertain to the therapist, his patient, and the social environment. Among the efforts to characterize these factors, some contributions concerning the therapist's attitude and the patient's personality structure and psychopathology would appear to promise or offer models for the trainee.

The desirable qualities and attitudes of the psychotherapist include his personal integrity, his intelligence, curiosity, and perceptiveness (especially a flair for empathizing with the psychological experiences of others), a talent for verbal communication, and the ability to look beyond the surface behavior of people, to understand rather than condemn them (Levine, 1942; Knight, 1952). Psychoanalysis has taught us that, along with these reasonable attributes and responses, we must reckon with the therapist's personal defenses and his countertransference reactions. Leo Berman (1949) characterized the totality of the psychoanalyst's emotional reactions as comprising an attitude of *dedication,* perhaps best seen under the fire of therapeutic crises and transference storms. The psychoanalyst, who tends to have the same kinds of reactions as do other people under similar stress, is better equipped to maintain a therapeutic effort through his having developed a greater variety of adaptations to different personalities; his responses are less intense or protracted and more flexible because he can work them through in self-analysis.

The capacity for dedication represents an ideal for the dy-

[97]

namic psychotherapist as well. Leo Stone (1961), writing about the psychoanalytic situation, similarly suggests that the basic attitude of the analyst is one of commitment, including the physician's unequivocal, sustained wish for his patient to get well. He contrasts the traditional physician's approach with its implied gratification of the patient's deep wishes for care and for the alleviation of guilt feelings—including the use of his authority, the "laying on of hands," the administering of medicines, the performance of surgery, and the mystery of his thinking and terminology to the lay person—with the emphasis in the psychoanalytic situation in which authoritarian advice is avoided, "contact" is made principally through speech, and the tendency is toward the exclusion of need fulfillment beyond the analyst's giving his understanding of the patient's emotional life. In terms of infantile fantasy the organic physician embodies the all-wise, all-powerful figure of the mother, who gives bodily care and sustains life, while the psychoanalyst represents the mother during the basic, temporary experiences of separation and deprivation which play an essential part in the infant's gradual achievement of self-object discrimination. The attitude of the psychotherapist moves between these two positions, according to the immediate needs and overall goals of the treatment.

Elizabeth R. Zetzel has emphasized the significance of the patient's personality and pathology as a factor limiting and defining the extent of therapeutic alliance. Crucial significance lies in the operative developmental level of object relations, especially the extent of achievement of self-object differentiation, the stability and autonomy of functions and structures, the availability in the ego of neutralized energy, the capacity to bear painful affects and the use of anxiety as a signal for defense. The psychotic or borderline patient who

[98]

has a poorly established personality organization and ill-defined ego boundaries, is self-preoccupied and mistrustful, and perceives the world largely in terms of reconstructive fantasy, may only develop a minimum rapport in treatment. This rapport might be a point of reliable contact or communication, and an indication that the therapist gratifies and means something to the patient. In order to appreciate different psychotherapeutic relationships and the patterns of therapy often associated with them, the resident needs experience in treating one or more patients representative of this borderline type, of the contrasting neurotic transference neurosis group, and also of those in a developmental crisis who fluctuate between borderline responses and predominantly normal or neurotic functioning.

Model Psychotherapeutic Patterns

Let us summarize these psychotherapeutic patterns. The first pertains to a chronic, exacerbated psychotic or borderline illness in an individual whose ego functions are impaired and whose attitude toward others is essentially narcissistic. When this hospitalized or ambulatory patient comes or is brought to us, he is entangled in a Gordian knot of social difficulties, involved in discord with his family, or tied in a symbiotic or parasitic relationship. Organic, psychosomatic, or hypochondriacal symptoms often color or dominate the picture. A slow progression in therapy may begin with abating the patient's efforts to withdraw or to deny any need for psychiatric treatment. The recapitulation of traumatic experiences and temporary symptomatic remissions alternate with demands for magical help and long, arid stretches of hypochondriacal, paranoid, or depressive complaining. Although suggestive indications of ego improvement and a better balance of drives and defenses appear sooner, it may take several years before substantial and sustained change occurs. This may be marked by a shift from narcissism to greater object appreciation, sometimes appearing in the psychotherapeutic relationship as a truer recognition of the therapist as a separate individual.

The second clinical model of psychotherapy would comprise the treatment of an acute emergency giving rise to anxiety, reactive depression or acting out, in a relatively healthy neurotic person who does not need to or cannot reasonably achieve profound changes in character. This patient readily forms a palpable, lively, and mainly positive transference. After assuring himself of the therapist's commitment to him (often by testing it out), while the intensity of his initial symptoms recedes, he begins to reexperience his conflicts in his impulses, thoughts and dreams, and to reenact them— creating a succession of minor crises—both within the psychotherapeutic relationship and, partly, acted out. As this behavior is clarified, he begins to deal more effectively with the precipitating causes of the original exigency. Initially, the dialogue of transference is the indication of therapeutic advance. Later, more stable improvement is correlated with the patient's increased objectivity, his more rapid and effective working through of repetitive conflicts, and his greater mastery of interpersonal problems.

Depending upon the ego strength and the emotional maturity of the patient, the pattern of psychotherapy of a developmental crisis partakes of both the shift from narcissism to greater object interest and the model of transference repetition of conflict. In addition, the therapeutic task is one of facilitating a psychobiological process with the goal of making a step in maturation, such as the achievement of the child-hood solution of the oedipal struggle, the goal of independence from the parents and a vocation for the adolescent, the goal of motherhood, etc. Often the stabilization of the crisis may be accomplished more readily than the clinical picture of chaotic turmoil or acute regression would lead one to expect.

The core of training in psychotherapy is supervised experience in the treatment of a few such well-selected patients. If a premature emphasis is placed upon very short-term therapy, the resident may not get past the early stages of establishing rapport, and is unlikely to acquire a feeling for dynamic movement, let alone maturational or structural change in his patients. He may miss out on experience with certain psychosomatic and borderline patients especially because of time limitations, since these patients require prolonged effort to help them overcome their initial resistance, and they are unusually vulnerable to separation trauma.

Models of Clinical Roles

The implied censure, pertinent or philistine, leveled at the psychotherapist—in the form of "Who will care for the great mass of mentally ill persons while you devote yourself to a few, relatively healthy ones?"—may be obviated in part by the understanding that residents are trained to serve flexibly in different clinical roles. These may be polarized as the formal function of therapist and the capacity of consultant. The therapist, who is the target of this criticism, concentrates upon the therapeutic relationship, whether it be with one patient or a group, and is pledged to the care of the patient for a long period, if necessary. In contrast, the consultant is relatively more concerned with the patient's total environment, as a result of which his commitment to the individual or group patient is more tentative. As a consultant the resident's primary task is to decipher the request for his assistance, which may not have come from the patient, and to answer it intelligently and, if possible, helpfully. He tries to establish rapport with the patient and with the significant people in his milieu (family, medical, cultural, educational, vocational, etc.). His diagnostic thinking includes them all. He reviews the range of feasible and indicated interventions and dispositions, considering their stabilizing, preventive, and corrective qualities. In this capacity he may undertake truly abbreviated therapy of limited scope, based upon achieving a sufficiently secure relationship without binding the patient to him, striving to stave off further pathological regression, selecting key problems to be dealt with, and encouraging favorable adaptive trends. The consultant role encompasses the handling of psychiatric emergencies, mental-hospital administrative psychotherapy, general hospital liaison psychiatry (Kahana, 1959), and a variety of social applications of psychotherapy, as in an affiliation with student health services and social agencies. Training as a consultant usually begins in the second, third, or fourth years of residency. In our experience *adaptive intervention* is especially useful as a curative agent to the psychiatric consultant.

MODELS OF CLINICAL SUPERVISION

The last models of psychotherapy to be considered are provided by clinical supervision. Among the various objectives of supervision, that of encouraging the resident's self-educative and self-corrective tendencies often develops through partial identifications with his instructors' skills, styles, and interests. The following appear foremost among the abilities thus personified: a synthesizing talent for absorbing details of the patient's past and ongoing behavior, and perceiving and formulating their interrelationship and essential significance for therapy; a facility for conceptualizing and vividly portraying the patient's personality in depth, preconsciously and unconsciously, from the recognized metapsychological viewpoints of psychic dynamics, energy distribution, structure, development, and adaptation; a command of techniques, with freedom to modify the rules and some originality; the capacity to keep alive one's own pleasure in the work despite its unusual strain; and special talents like the gift for visualizing "the child in the adult," a sure feeling for the transference, aptitude in translating nonverbal communications, and proficiency in treating dependent, delinquent, depressed, blocked, withdrawn, hypersensitive or very hostile patients.

If we look ahead, it appears likely that the effective applications of psychotherapy will continue to grow in scope, and that observations, theories, and techniques will become better defined, as more needed people enter the various professional disciplines which have begun to take an active role in the enormous field of mental illness. While some economy of time and effort is afforded by evolving teaching models such as those we have considered—models of therapeutic aims, principles, relationships, patterns, and styles of practice, and of basic theory—the length of training in this skill for the psychiatric resident will probably not shorten if his formative experience is to consist of more than a series of evaluations, introductions, and broken-off treatments.

Psychoanalytic Theory and the Teaching of Dynamic Psychiatry

RUDOLPH M. LOEWENSTEIN, M.D.

W HEN DR. GRETE BIBRING invited me to participate in this symposium, I felt honored but also puzzled. What perplexed me was the subject: "Can psychiatry be taught? A reappraisal of the goals and techniques in the teaching of psychiatry." I reacted to it, not unnaturally, by a somewhat agonizing reappraisal of my personal position on this question. Was it possible, I asked myself, that I was a fraud in believing for many years that I had actually taught some people psychoanalysis, or psychotherapy, or even psychiatry? After some soul searching, I reassured myself that I had not been an imposter. But a certain doubt persisted, and still does, for I am not sure that I know precisely what is meant by dynamic psychiatry. I presume, however, that, as its name indicates, it takes into account the effects of unconscious psychic forces on mental illness. At any rate, I consoled myself with the thought that one might be equally hard put to define psychoanalysis— or surgery, for that matter.

After a brief turmoil, I was left with the challenge to clarify some of my ideas concerning how an analyst's knowledge can contribute to that of a psychiatric resident. I do not know whether I will be able to meet this challenge in a fruitful way, especially since my activity has been limited chiefly to the teaching of psychoanalytic candidates, with the exception of a few years during which I taught psychiatric residents at Yale. The problem then seemed to reduce itself to a few more circumscribed questions. How much can be taught by any teacher or by books? What cannot be taught and thus must be learned by experience, if at all? It is evident that the particular setup of the institution where residents work will play a considerable role in what can or cannot be taught them within a much wider training program.

Leaving aside the important factor of the talent and intuition of a given resident, I wonder in what way analytic theory, or what part of it, can be usefully conveyed to the psychiatric resident, and what can be gained from it. Let me describe a clinical case which made a deep impression on me when I was attending a course in psychiatry as a medical student. I cite it here because a psychiatric resident may be faced by a similar case at any time in his work. This example is concerned with the relation of psychoanalytic theory to the diagnosis of psychoses.

Dr. Bonhoeffer, then head of the Department of Psychiatry at the University of Berlin, presented a young woman who complained of fear of sharp objects, particularly of knives, lest she might kill her husband. The question was whether the patient was schizophrenic or obsessive-compulsive, and whether she should be sent home or kept in the hospital. A young resident was entrusted with the task of examining her and of making a diagnosis and recommendation. Although he was extremely well versed in psychoanalytic theory (and was to later become a famous psychoanalyst), he obviously had had relatively little clinical experience. This young man recommended that the patient be discharged and sent home insofar as he considered her case one of obsessive-compulsive neurosis. Some days later, the patient was back in the hospital: she actually had killed her husband.

Perhaps this erroneous diagnosis had been unavoidable at that stage of the patient's illness. On the other hand, an experienced clinician unfamiliar with psychoanalytic theory would have been better equipped to detect an incipient acute schizophrenic episode in this patient than would an inexperienced psychiatric resident who had excellent knowledge of it. Experienced clinicians make use of many signs they perceive in patients, signs which have found no place as yet in our theoretical considerations.

Is psychoanalytic theory then of little or no value in matters of differential diagnosis between psychosis and neurosis? In the case mentioned, one could see a homicidal impulse being warded off by inner defenses. This is a state of affairs common to both psychosis and obsessive-compulsive neurosis; the difference between them can be inferred from the outcome of the conflict. Psychoanalytic theory speaks of a difference in relative power or strength between impulse and defense. This quantitative formulation is a statement made after the fact, and has no predictive and hence no diagnostic value, unless a knowledge of the patient's history permits some inferences based on the outcome of past conflicts.

In a general way, the existence of intrapsychic conflicts does not by itself differentiate psychoses from neuroses, one neurosis from another, or even mental illness from mental health. Freud (1911) described the situation as follows, when discussing the mechanism of paranoia in his classic paper on the Schreber case.

> We have hitherto been dealing with the father-complex, which was the dominant element . . . and with the wishful phantasy round which the illness centred. But in all of this there is nothing characteristic of the form of disease known as paranoia, nothing that might not be found (and that has not in fact been found) in other kinds of neuroses. The distinctive character of paranoia (or of dementia paranoides) must be sought for elsewhere—namely, in the particular form assumed by the symptoms; and we shall expect to find that this is determined, not by the nature of the complexes themselves, but by the mechanisms by which the symptoms are formed or by which repression is brought about [p. 59].

Equally pertinent is Freud's statement in a letter addressed in 1915 to Karl Abraham, concerning the psychological difference between obsessional neurosis and melancholia:

> I will only lay stress on two points: that you do not emphasize enough the essential part of my hypothesis, i.e. the topographical consideration in it, the regression of the libido and the abandoning of the unconscious cathexis, and that instead you put sadism and anal-erotism in the foreground as the final explanation. Anal-erotism, castration complexes, etc., are ubiquitous sources of excitation which must have their share in *every* clinical picture. One time this is made from them, another time that. Naturally we have the task of ascertaining what is made from them, but the explanation of the disorder can only be found in the mechanism—considered dynamically, topographically and economically. [Cited by Jones, 1955, p. 329.]

[107]

Thus in the case of schizophrenic disorder, the role of the mechanism of projection is predominant, and the relationship to the objects is deeply disturbed. Freud (1911) described it in terms of a regression of the libido to a narcissistic stage. At a later date Freud (1924) stressed that the relevant pathogenic conflict in a psychosis is between the ego and outside reality, whereas neuroses are based on conflicts between the ego and the id.

More recently Hartmann (1953) expanded the psychoanalytic theory of schizophrenia in metapsychological terms. He emphasized that disturbances originating in autonomous ego functions, such as thought disorders and disturbed object relations, contribute in turn to the impairment of the defensive functions of the ego.

To recapitulate, I am convinced that in diagnosing an incipient psychosis, good clinical experience by itself is more useful than familiarity with analytic theory alone. The optimum, of course, is to have both, each supplementing and enriching the other. Knowledge of the psychoanalytic theory is essential for understanding one's patients' disorders on a broad basis, and even for learning, that is, for acquiring clinical experience. In the latter situation, theoretical formulations may perform the task of markers or pointers to clarify the topography in uncharted or little-known territory.

At this point we might reflect in a more general manner upon the reach and the implications of some theoretical propositions in analysis. One can examine them from the viewpoint of what type of statements they make in relation to observable data. I should like to cite the introductory paragraphs of a paper in which I deal with this subject (Loewenstein, 1965).

In psychoanalysis, as in any other scientific endeavor, the relationship between data of observation and theoretical propositions or concepts is highly complex. Some underlying hypotheses or theoretical assumptions, whether explicitly formulated or implicit in the mind of the investigator, are necessary to make an observational datum out of the formless mass of perceived phenomena. In each individual analysis there is an interplay between observation and the application of some theoretical assumption or hypothesis, without which the observational data would simply remain in a state of chaos (Hartmann, Kris, and Loewenstein, 1953). In psychoanalysis the essential, explicitly formulated hypothesis underlying observational data is that apparently meaningless psychic phenomena, such as dreams, neurotic symptoms or random thoughts, are determined by unconscious psychic processes exerting dynamic effects on the conscious mind.

In psychoanalysis there are propositions which consist of generalizations based upon observable data or in extrapolations derived from them. Some generalizations serve to group various data together and to delineate them from others. An example of such a generalization appears when we put together some psychic tendencies on one side of conflict situations, and some other kind of tendencies on the other side of such conflicts. This classification may be further generalized and conceptualized as the conflict between forces of instinctual drives in opposition to forces of the ego. Another type of generalization is the statement that oedipal conflicts in childhood are not findings limited to some neurotic individuals but are ubiquitous and characteristic of human development in general. Extrapolations of various kinds are propositions referred to phenomena not obviously observable in the data. They are used to describe the data in a more

[109]

satisfactory way. One type of extrapolation is the reconstruction of early developmental stages arrived at from observing disturbances of present-day functions. It is obvious that the examples given here do not exhaust all the inferences and deductions drawn from psychoanalytic data of observation. Most if not all of these generalizations and extrapolations can be validated or invalidated by the use of the very method thanks to which they were arrived at—the method of psychoanalysis. However, there exist in psychoanalysis a number of other propositions which can never be either confirmed or invalidated by the psychoanalytic method proper. They can only be formulated or discarded on the basis of their usefulness and inner consistency. These propositions are the explanatory concepts and constructs which form the psychoanalytic metapsychology (Freud, 1915; Hartmann, 1927 and 1959; Rapaport and Gill, 1959; Rapaport, 1960). Metapsychological propositions made psychoanalysis into a scientific psychology based on models equivalent to those of other natural sciences.

Psychoanalysis, thus, has theories referring to phenomena that can be observed in the present or in the future. And it has theories, or it uses concepts, referring to phenomena that can never be directly observed by the psychoanalytic method. Force, or energy, be it physical or psychic, or the mental apparatus and its component systems—the ego, id and superego—can never be observed as such. In contradistinction, a reconstructed unconscious wish or fantasy, or the action of unconscious defense mechanisms, if not observed directly, is inferred from its impact on observable material and, what is essential, is built on the model of their observable and conscious counterparts. These inferred phenomena are thus *homologous* to the phenomena from which their existence was inferred. The inferred existence, for instance, of a libid-

[110]

inal drive or of an ego refers to another category of assumed phenomena that are *heterologous* to the observable phenomena which they serve to explain or to describe. In spite of the "distance" separating the data and these propositions, the latter are nevertheless not totally independent of the former. There must exist some *congruence between the data and these propositions in order for these to be fruitful.*

Psychoanalysis uses and needs both types of propositions in its theory, in its method, and in its practical applications. However, the relative value of these two types of propositions varies, depending upon whether we consider psychoanalysis as a body of knowledge, as a method of investigation, or as a therapeutic procedure [pp. 38-40].

I mentioned in the preceding quoted material that one of the characteristics of psychoanalytic theoretical formulations is their broad basis. By this I meant that they apply not only to a given patient in dealing with one particular clinical problem, but that they also have general validity in dealing with all patients and all kinds of clinical situations during therapeutic as well as diagnostic work. For instance, by using such terms as "the unconscious" or "the id," the psychiatrist's attention will be directed toward the many and varied clinical phenomena in his patient which are implicitly subsumed under these concepts. Or in remembering the concept of transference, he will be reminded of the fact that the patient's reactions to him during treatment can be understood as repetitions of older, unconscious reactions to a person in the patient's past.

Let us consider the example mentioned at the beginning: the relative strength of the aggressive impulse or the relative weakness of the ego defenses in schizophrenia. At first sight such an explanation seems of little value, and yet it has both general and specific import. Such quantitative evaluation, imprecise and vague as it may appear, can decide what type of therapeutic procedure may or may not be used in particular cases. This economic approach also has an influence on our ideas and actions concerned with the prevention of neuroses and with the upbringing of children.

We have presupposed here that the psychiatrist performs an implicit translation from the general and abstract to the individual and concrete. This translation has a grammatical connotation as well: an impersonal statement in theory becomes a personal statement in the doctor-patient relationship. I referred above to phenomena which are *homologous* to those from which their existence was inferred. They alone can be translated into propositions enunciated in the first person. To give an example: the concept of transference resistance is used by the therapist in such a way as to enable the patient to express his awareness that resentment toward the therapist is a repetition of similar feelings toward his father.

This part of the psychiatrist's work, namely, the task of translating general theoretical formulations into concrete personal statements, is not an easy one at all. Often he falters because such a translation evokes some personal reaction in himself. Medical students not uncommonly are affected by hypochondriacal fears of the illnesses they study. Those who study psychiatric disorders incline rather to the opposite, to deny the possibility of having anything in common with such patients. Whereas the bodily illness is an external danger, the emotional disorder is an internal threat reminding us of similar reactions in our own past, which we are proud to have overcome. To confront these disorders, and to deal with them, requires an amount of empathy that may threaten the psychiatrist with loss of control. But the ability to translate the general and abstract into the concrete and individual is bound up with his capacity for empathy.

What practical conclusions with respect to the teaching of dynamic psychiatry can be drawn from the preceding remarks? One conclusion seems obvious at first sight: that a personal analysis of the psychiatric resident will diminish his fear of empathizing with the patient's unconscious reactions, and will give him a first-hand experience of the empirical basis for some concepts and theoretical propositions. This is indeed of inestimable value to a psychiatrist. However, the personal analysis is unfortunately not the answer to *all* problems. In the specialized training of psychoanalysts, a didactic analysis is accompanied by formal instruction in theory, clinic, and technique. Such training is even more necessary in the teaching of dynamic psychiatry. A young psychiatrist will be all too prone to regard the conditions under which a psychoanalysis is conducted as the model for any therapeutic situation. This tendency can lead to unfortunate results. The psychoanalytic setup and some technical rules are valid for analysis, and for analysis alone. They are not useful, indeed may be harmful, if applied to a different kind of treatment in certain types of cases. I am referring here, for example, to patients for whom psychoanalysis is contraindicated or not advisable under given circumstances. For example, in a psychoanalytic treatment we tend to emphasize the analysis of *all* transference reactions; not so in a psychotherapy, where the therapeutic use of positive transference is much more pronounced than the analytic reduction of it.

Although psychoanalytic theory has never been completely systematized and is not a closed system, one cannot arbitrarily remove parts of it without potentially disrupting the meaning

[113]

of the whole. But this does not mean that the whole of theory must be taught, especially outside a psychoanalytic institute. The question in my opinion is not how much or how little psychoanalytic theory is to be taught, but rather how it is to be done.

The teaching of psychoanalytic theory should thus be divided into two areas, with particular attention to its place within the framework of psychiatric training:

(1) The theory of psychoanalytic technique, encompassing the considerations against a use of certain technical rules in various psychotherapeutic procedures.

(2) The teaching of clinical theory and of metapsychology, aiming not so much at completeness as at correlation with observational data. It should emphasize the clinical observations which have led to our theoretical propositions, and show the way back from theory to the concrete and specific.

Discussion

Dr. TARTAKOFF: The discipline of psychoanalysis is to some extent burdened by the fact that it attempts to fulfill the requirements of a general psychology at the same time that it serves as a method of treatment. Dr. Loewenstein has told us that psychoanalysis uses and needs different types of propositions and that their importance varies, depending on whether we consider psychoanalysis as a body of knowledge, a method of investigation, or a therapeutic procedure. He says: "Some underlying hypotheses or theoretical assumptions, whether explicitly formulated or implicit in the mind of the investigator, are necessary to make an observational datum out of the formless mass of perceived phenomena" (p. 109).

If this is true for a general theory, it has proved to be essential for our clinical theory as well. Without models and a theory, how could the inexperienced resident bring order to (1) the chaotic eruptions of emotions characteristic of certain acute psychotic states, (2) the extreme, although limited, disorganization of the patient in a developmental crisis, (3) the

Drs. Maxwell Gitelson, Lawrence S. Kubie, Gregory Rochlin, and Elizabeth R. Zetzel delivered prepared discussions by invitation.

Drs. Douglas D. Bond, Arthur F. Valenstein, Ralph J. Kahana, and Rudolf M. Loewenstein took part in the general discussion.

decompensation of severe psychosomatic conditions, or even (4) the inappropriate repetitions of the neurotic.

The resident psychiatrist whose career commitment—for whatever reasons—brings him into close contact with psychopathology, would flounder without a theoretical framework. In fact, he would be forced to begin where Kraepelin and his followers left off, classifying types of mental illness. Therefore, although we may look ahead with some degree of consternation to what the future holds, with its emphasis on molecular biology, we may also look back with considerable gratification to the giant steps which have been taken in the past 65 years.

DR. GITELSON: It is true that what we call dynamic psychology is possible in the hands of specially talented people; that such people can give extensive psychotherapy directed toward producing a degree of insight, a degree of resolution of conflicts, and a degree of ego control. Dynamic psychotherapy is in fact a highly modified derivative of psychoanalysis, directed toward limited therapeutic goals. At best it can be very good; but not infrequently it is wild analysis.

Another question was touched on, that of commitment and dedication. I think these are noble terms—at times I think of myself as committed, and at times I think of myself as dedicated. But this is unearned increment, because primarily I am *interested*. I cannot remember the time when I was not interested in other human beings—although there were times when I was scared to death of them. So, commitment and dedication—yes. True, these qualities become a part of us, but primarily we have an operating interest in terms of a problem to solve, in terms of an adaptational problem, not only for the patient but for the encounter with the patient. I suppose some of you would prefer to refer to this encounter as "transference," but I think the word "encounter" is more expressive of the total relationship.

I was struck this morning by the assumption that our medical students and residents would be better off if they learned about the generalities of life by studying the behavioral sciences than if they were simply given instruction in psychoanalysis. It occurred to me (and it was mentioned as the final spearhead of Dr. Loewenstein's address) that psychoanalysis as a science provides what we need and is inclusive of what is proposed in behavioral-science instruction. In our newer and broadening conceptions of the holistic aspects of psychoanalysis, we inevitably are confronted with the necessity of considering everything which belongs to man. Psychoanalysis, as a general psychology, provides us with a bridge to the behavioral sciences. At the same time it serves to link all the behavioral sciences, and enables us to make use of these sciences in our clinical work, to which we as psychiatrists are committed. That brings me back to the question of training residents. In such places as Boston where there is an outstanding institute, and at other places where there are institutes which may or may not be outstanding, the institute provides a magnetic point, a focus for the training of psychiatric residents. In these places there is a tendency, no matter how one attempts to avoid it, to remain fixed to the goal and purpose of psychoanalysis, with the consequence that there is a greater and greater tendency to confuse the teaching of so-called dynamic psychiatry with what I would call amateur analysis or wild analysis.

There is every reason to teach as much of basic psychoanalytic theory and psychopathology as the resident can absorb— this against a truly rich background of clinical, descriptive,

[117]

and diagnostic psychiatry. When it comes to management and psychotherapy, it is necessary and possible to teach this material psychoanalytically, but in its own terms. I conduct analytic treatment without a single reference to a technical word or a theoretical concept, and I believe it is possible to teach the "sense and meaning" of a human being in this way.

DR. TARTAKOFF: It is not quite clear to me whether or not Dr. Gitelson believes that psychotherapy with limited goals is valid or invalid. It is further unclear whether or not he is saying psychotherapy can best be done by the analyst, and that therefore one should not attempt interim psychotherapy. I think this is one of the questions some of the others may want to pick up. His second point is a very interesting one. As a general psychology, psychoanalysis can be used in training residents by applying it individually to each resident and teaching him as much as he is ready or able to learn.

DR. KUBIE: The term "dynamic psychiatry" is in constant use. Every once in a while, therefore, it becomes appropriate to ask ourselves what it means. As with all terms, it has a history, a review of which would probably show that it arose in protest against something static and descriptive. Perhaps we can agree that it implied an effort to find explanations of psychological events in the interactions among prior psychological experiences and their after-images, without resorting to what Adolf Meyer used to call "neurologizing tautologies."

The word "dynamic" might also represent a whole chain of successive proclamations of emancipation for psychology—the first from theology and philosophy, the second from neurosensory physiology. The third involves the expansion of the whole field of psychology to include considerations of unconscious as well as conscious levels of experience. Certainly then, the term has served a hopeful purpose, even if it lacks clarity.

This lack of clarity leads to a period of groping which we should welcome, since the assumption that we know what the words mean has blocked any exploration of the concept. Even today the term can mislead us into assuming that we have achieved the goal of creating a dynamic psychology, while it obscures the fact that this is still an unrealized hope.

In any science, "dynamic" implies the transition from description to explanation, something which is always difficult, but hardest of all in psychology. The dilemma is an old one. Usually we fool ourselves about this by pretending that merely the refinement of descriptions automatically gives them explanatory values. Whether one is a layman in the street or a highly specialized technician, these verbal traps are difficult to avoid. The layman has no hesitation in talking as though he can explain psychological changes in purely psychological terms. And we, the professionals, forget all we know about post-hoc or propterhoc fallacies and attribute causal significance to sequences of events, forgetting that although sequences make causal relationships possible they can never prove them. Nor do they even make them probable until the uniqueness, adequacy, necessity and invariability of the sequence has been established. Similarly, we allow such descriptively useful abstractions as id and superego to become anthropomorphic entities, homunculi within us, power-packs of independent and mythical energetic processes. Or, we formulate dynamic psychology solely in terms of motives and purposes, whether these operate consciously, or on preconscious or unconscious levels. Certainly, even as descriptions, our concepts of dynamic purposes must include unconscious

[119]

as well as conscious purposes, and conscious or unconscious conflicts among irreconcilable purposes. But none of this is enough to justify our calling it dynamic. Psychology cannot become dynamic until we can clarify the psychological mechanisms by which purposes are implemented, by which they can be internally blocked, and by which a resolution of internal obstacles can be achieved—as well as the mechanisms determining the pathological symptoms which form as by-products of these struggles and the secondary and tertiary consequences of these symptoms as well.

My personal conviction is that the vital and central fact in human psychology is that *only preconscious processes are dynamic*. Therefore, when Freud turned his thoughts away from his early formulation of the preconscious system, psychoanalytic psychology temporarily ceased to be a dynamic psychology. (The term preconscious had almost dropped out of the literature until Ernst Kris resurrected it. I am sure that he would have carried this process of resurrection further but for his untimely death.) If this is true, then we must teach our residents not merely the nature of psychopathogenic unconscious conflicts, or the conscious symbolic representations of those conflicts in symptomatic behavior, but also the flow of preconscious processing which is the stuff of human living. This is dynamic psychiatry, and the problem of how to teach it is the same, whether we try to teach it to the medical student, to the psychiatric resident, or to a patient.

When we attempt to teach this subject to anyone, we trigger in him echoes of his own problems and his counterphobic defenses against them. How then can the teaching of dynamic psychiatry be achieved without involving the student in some form of therapeutic experience? It is my conviction that such an approach is not only impossible, but actually wrong. We shy away from this because we are frightened by the implications of the stark fact that in psychiatry learning is nothing unless it is also a therapeutic experience. (Some day we will have to face up to the fact that the same principle holds for all education from the kindergarten on up.) This is one reason why supervision in small groups is one of our best educational instruments, i.e., because its very nature is simultaneously a process of group therapy and of group learning. It is also the best preparation for subsequent individual therapy, and this is how I have used it at the Sheppard and Enoch Pratt Hospital for the last six years.

As individuals, the rate at which we mature depends partly upon our willingness to accept in our own lives the complex and maturing experiences of living. As psychiatrists, our rate of growth depends upon the rate at which patients can change. As clinicians, therapists, and students, we grow up by living with patients through the slow process of change—and this we cannot hurry. We can condense and summarize this process and describe these changes in books, but we cannot rush the process of change itself. So, too, as teachers we achieve maturity at a rate limited by the rate at which our students change. The maturational process in the student, in the teacher, and in the patient takes time.

Let me say finally that we will never solve these problems until we shake off the dead hand of the past, and reduce the role which traditionalism still plays in psychiatric teaching. We will have to face the fact that it is medical malpractice to start the young psychiatrist off by confronting him with psychotic patients in a psychiatric hospital. He should start with the infant, then progress through the toddler stage, the latency period, puberty, and early adolescence to the neuroses of adult life on medical and surgical wards, moving from that

[121]

base of experience to the psychiatric outpatient department, and only then to the psychiatric hospital. It is essential to have some mastery of the neurotic process, some experience of it as a developing process, before attempting to accept the challenge of the psychoses. The many reasons for this are presented in detail in my paper (Kubie, 1964), "Traditionalism in Psychiatry." These are a few of the stepping stones toward education in a dynamic psychiatry.

DR. TARTAKOFF: I appreciate Dr. Kubie's pointing out the absence of a definition for this Symposium. It is reassuring that we do not have to come to a definition today, but can leave that to the panels that follow. However, I would like to ask whether Dr. Kubie and Dr. Gitelson are not making somewhat similar points, although they approach them by different routes. Dr. Gitelson emphasizes that we should try to teach a resident only what he can learn, and that in the process of teaching, we should be very aware both of what he can absorb and of what may deter him from being able to assimilate knowledge at a certain period in his development. Dr. Kubie carries this point further by a strong statement that resident teaching should be a therapeutic process and also be recognized as one. Perhaps we should ask: Is teaching always a therapeutic process but not recognized as such? Is this the emphasis Dr. Kubie means? We shall continue with the planned discussion, and then let both participants answer for themselves.

DR. ROCHLIN: As I review my thoughts, I find that they are directed more at the teachers than at the residents. First, a little about students. When we speak of teaching dynamic psychiatry, we must bear in mind that we are concerned with a resident who is not simply resistant. Unlike the medical student we were describing this morning, the resident is different. He has committed himself to psychiatry. In fact, as we have all experienced, he is often overcommitted, in contrast to the medical student. Moreover, the resident is by no means ignorant; in fact, he is usually a very well-informed man as well as being well educated. The milieu is as important for the resident as for the medical student. A great deal depends on the working milieu the resident is offered and on how he responds to it. The psychiatric resident in a general hospital is presented with a very different milieu than is his counterpart in a mental hospital such as the one in which I work, the Massachusetts Mental Health Center. In granting that there are certain advantages in a general hospital, I want also to call attention to the fact that the chief of service or the chief of the hospital is a clinical administrator, and that his bias is important to the kind of shadow he casts on the staff and on the resident.

What is this shadow falling on the resident that I consider to be a problem? It is primarily the tyranny of technique. I see the physician as tyrannized by the need for technique and clinical management—not that the circumstances fail to demand both. Nor is the chief of service of a hospital unaware that these are his obligations, in the sense that he has certain clinical, managerial, and administrative problems that must be resolved. I feel that he must guard against this tyranny, however, because he is also the teacher, also the ruler of the staff, and also the model for the residents—if we are going to talk about models. He must guard against the fact that his position requires him to do certain things, behave in a certain way in relationship to certain patients. But it is seldom the resident's job to take similar action. It is my impression that

[123]

the resident-in-training is making inordinate demands for techniques in both the treatment of patients and their clinical management. I think a teacher must be very wary not to be swayed by such demands on the part of residents. These doctors are fumbling, learning, and trying to pick their way through the difficulties attendant on the fact that they find very sick patients present.

There is a tendency to place such demands ahead of the need to acquire an understanding of people. The residents demand the technique of how to manage people, how to deal with them, instead of seeking an understanding of these people. I say people rather than patients because I think it is proper to keep in mind that a good deal of what the psychiatrist does (i.e., the one who is teaching dynamic psychiatry) has to include relatives. Here again I am not speaking about a technique of handling relatives, but about understanding the fact that we are dealing with families of people. Neither as teacher nor as resident can one isolate oneself in a one-to-one patient relationship in a hospital (unless the hospital is especially designed for this purpose) without making life either a caricature of analysis or subservient to psychiatry.

To Dr. Rosenbaum's statement that the teacher of psychoanalysis is not the same person who practices psychoanalysis, I should like to comment that this is the way it should be. I do not feel that I should come into the hospital as a psychoanalyst and conduct myself as a psychoanalyst there. I think that it is appropriate neither to the hospital nor to what the resident needs to be taught. Too often this happens, and it should be considered a hazard an analyst must guard against.

In respect to the same problem, I would like to pick up a comment of Dr. Bond's. He says that one must show what one does. Certainly, teaching should utilize demonstration and should guard against the tendency to become a strictly supervisory method. The teacher is prone to spend much time supervising, without seeing live material, so that his clinical experience becomes a vicarious one through residents. I doubt if this is really clinical teaching. In turn, such an approach supports unwittingly the tendency to fulfill the demand for technique. The result is to invite more of those technical demands that the resident-in-training naturally will ask for.

Dr. Gitelson has pointed out that some analysts have felt that if they conduct themselves primarily as teachers (and not so much as analysts) they do not become psychoanalysts. I suggest that they won't. As analysts, we should not try to teach psychoanalysis to residents. That is not what they need, nor what they should have; moreover, analysis should not be confused with dynamic psychiatry. Another consideration is that psychoanalysts find themselves in a unique position as teachers, unlike teachers in other fields of medicine. A surgeon teaches his resident surgery, a pediatrician, pediatrics; but what does a psychoanalyst teach his residents? He does not teach them psychoanalysis. He teaches clinical psychiatry, and in this he differs from his colleagues in other fields of medicine. I do not agree with Dr. Loewenstein that the whole problem is restricted to the question: how should psychoanalysis be taught? To me, "how" is not so much a problem as "who" should be taught it. Dr. Kahana has listed in detail the rough schedules, rates, and strains with which the resident is burdened. His emphasis is on the technique. In the course of his paper, Dr. Knight has pointed out aims that are supportive to psychoanalytic understanding. Those objectives that Dr. Gitelson has proposed are related to the duration of active therapy, or brief therapy, or long-term therapy, and to advice on technique.

It seems to me that this approach once more furnishes a resident with *methods* rather than with *meaning,* the means rather than the ends. For many reasons, I do not regret the lack of a particular handbook of principles and procedures for a resident to follow. I have the impression that an adherence to a handbook of principles would be at the cost of understanding. I am struck by my own experience with the most advanced residents, men in their third and fourth years of residency, in child psychiatry. It is a rare individual who in less than six months of the first year of child psychiatry can feel comfortable with a child's infantile material. Remember, he is a man who not only has been taught carefully and been supervised well, but also is bright and capable. Moreover, he has been trained for at least two or three years before he comes to us. The less he demands technique, the more advanced his understanding and his skill.

DR. ZETZEL: Several speakers have already raised questions about the meaning of the term "dynamic psychiatry." In my own psychiatric and analytic training there was no such discipline as "dynamic psychiatry." On the one hand, there was psychoanalysis, which I studied at the London Institute of Psychoanalysis; on the other, there was academic psychiatry, which I learned at the Maudsley Hospital. It appeared to me then that never the twain should meet. The language we used and the goals we envisaged were very different. After living in this bilingual world for more than 10 years, I returned to this country some 15 years ago. It was only at that time that I first heard the words "dynamic psychiatry." When I began teaching at the Boston Institute of Psychoanalysis,

[126]

my geographical transposition posed no particular problem of adjustment. When, however, I began to teach psychiatry to residents and medical students in the Boston area, I was faced with quite a different situation. This I will try to describe as briefly as possible.

The first impact on me of assuming my presumed identity as a teacher of "dynamic psychiatry" was that of considerable consternation and confusion. The term "dynamic psychiatry" seemed to imply the substitution of psychoanalytic reconstructions for the teaching of formal clinical psychiatry. This, I felt, was often inappropriate and in addition inadequate with respect to diagnostic appraisal and treatment goals. There had been, I believe, a premature attempt to achieve a union between psychiatry and psychoanalysis, allowing the latter substantially to replace traditional description and diagnostic formulation. In other words, I agree very strongly with Dr. Loewenstein's position, to the effect that a knowledge of psychoanalysis cannot replace clinical experience in psychiatry, which is essential for all future psychiatrists. Psychiatric skills are not conferred by psychoanalytic training, however much this training may enrich and sharpen many techniques relevant to clinical psychiatry.

I believe that we still make some errors in this particular area. There is a tendency to think that psychoanalytic training almost automatically equips the student to be a competent psychiatrist, a good diagnostician, and a good nonanalytic psychotherapist. There could be no greater error. I believe this misconception has disadvantageously influenced the positive impact of psychoanalysis on academic psychiatry. In this context, I personally feel that the term "dynamic psychiatry" is essentially to be regarded as a euphemism. It is, after all, only a more general and less specific term than is

[127]

"psychoanalytic psychiatry." We have not heard one word today under the heading "dynamic psychiatry" which has not
in fact referred to the applications of psychoanalysis, both
the method and the theory, in the teaching of medical students and the training of psychiatrists. All that has been said
has been based on the major assumption of psychoanalysis,
not only in respect to the body of knowledge taught, but also
in respect to our understanding of the psychological problems of the student at every level of training.

One important general problem which emerged this morning and has been underlined this afternoon concerns itself
with the distinction between psychoanalysis as a body of
knowledge and psychoanalysis as a specific therapeutic method. The first concerns an increasingly comprehensive psychology, equally applicable to normal development and to pathological conditions. This body of knowledge is more or less objective and has been more or less validated. The second concerns the method, that is, traditional psychoanalysis, by means
of which most of this knowledge was originally acquired. I
would like to compare the body of objective knowledge and
the specific clinical techniques to parallel features of the
learning process at a more general level. Dr. Bond, quoting
Kris, has remarked that learning is facilitated either by positive transference or by an appeal to the intellect. This differentiation leads to the recognition of two important and
different aspects of learning and maturation. On the one
hand, that which is taken in passively and integrated in Dr.
Kubie's preconscious part of the mind may be related to positive transference. On the other hand, that which is approached actively, using secondary process thinking and conscious
memory, leading to active mastery, appeals to the intellect.
This type of learning must be contrasted with that which is

passively absorbed by intuition or preconscious integration.

We constantly swing back and forth between these two modes of learning. They are particularly relevant to the learning process in psychiatry. As Dr. Kahana has mentioned, the young resident is passively exposed to a great deal of material with considerable emotional impact at a time when he has few, if any, techniques for mastery. Moreover, at the beginning of his training he has no significant objective conceptual framework on which to fall back for reassurance. For this reason I think it desirable that the beginning resident be given adequate opportunities to use his mind. Some understanding of descriptive psychiatry and some introduction to conceptual theory partially counteract the abrupt exposure to and overwhelming impact of the immediate clinical material. This he is not prepared to handle effectively, without help in the beginning stages of his psychiatric education.

This emotional impact is of course essential and can lead to the kind of experiences Dr. Kubie has defined as "therapeutic." These I would prefer to call "maturational." Incidentally, I would also regard psychotherapy as a maturational experience, since to some degree important maturational steps must always occur at a preconscious level. Emotional growth implies both regression and progression, which are integral to the learning process. I do not believe that this type of experience can replace a personal psychoanalysis. Nevertheless, it is an experience which, like the resolution of early conflicts, or identity formation in adolescence, does combine some regressive features with subsequent active mastery which is part of the final definitive process of maturation.

In considering psychotherapy, other than psychoanalysis, in relation to psychiatric training, I think we should recognize that we have not yet achieved a theory of the therapeutic process on a par with our theory of psychoanalysis itself. This should be abundantly clear from the different points of view and the amount of disagreement that have been expressed today. If we are in agreement that psychoanalysis itself is a relatively young discipline, we would have to say that psychotherapy has not yet reached the adolescent identity crisis which Dr. Gitelson described in a recent paper. I do believe, however, that the emergence of the crisis in psychoanalysis is highly relevant, not only to the future of psychoanalysis but also to the growth and integration within our conceptual framework of the new therapeutic techniques, such as those that have come out of the Beth Israel Hospital in recent years.

It is essential in this endeavor to differentiate between post-hoc explanations of a therapeutic intervention which has been accomplished, and our ongoing supervision of psychiatrists in training. As Dr. Loewenstein has indicated, it is one thing to explain an accomplished fact (many successful therapeutic maneuvers could be described as successful adaptive intervention at the most general level), but it is quite another to use one's knowledge of both theory and practice before the fact—to use it in a diagnostic evaluation which includes implicit predictions. Therefore, I fully agree with Dr. Loewenstein's emphasis on the importance of training in clinical psychiatry. It is my feeling, however, that a comprehensive education in the broad framework of psychoanalytic knowledge as a developmental psychology is highly advantageous. From this point of view I must disagree with Dr. Loewenstein on a specific clinical issue. I believe that psychoanalytic psychiatry stands today in a markedly different position from that which prevailed when he was a medical student, or when I started in psychiatric training at the Maudsley Hospital in 1938. In respect to diagnostic evaluation, we have carried our developmental hypothesis beyond the type of instinctual classification which dominated psychiatric evaluation at that time. We are often now in a position to make a more accurate evaluation of the difference between primitive and mature modes of thought, perception, and feeling, and of their diagnostic implications. Our understanding of object relations, though still subject to controversy, is also highly relevant. I believe, for example, that a contemporary psychoanalytic psychiatrist might be able to evaluate patients like the one with the knife phobia in terms of evidence of primitive mode of thought, the loss of capacity for positive object relations, or the regressive perception of danger (which Dr. Max Schur described), and thus make it possible to see the patient as an incipient psychotic rather than an obsessional neurotic.

In summary: psychiatric training epitomizes the two poles of the learning process, passive reception and active mastery. Training which emphasizes the one to the exclusion of the other does not further individual growth and maturation. Despite individual differences in respect to aptitudes at both extremes, the training programs should provide ample opportunities to further both types of learning at every level.

* * *

DR. BOND: Recently Anna Freud described three major sources of a medical student's desire to enter medicine. The first, she said, was curiosity, the normal curiosity that every child has if it has not been dampened. This form of curiosity is a fine motive for entering medicine, and frequently these students become researchers. The second source lies in the child's reac-

[131]

tion formation to his own sadism, and these people are likely to be the "carers," those who want to take care of people. The third source lies in the need of some to prove their potency and the magical ability to make the ill rise and walk. These are very important human motives, but I think it is also important to realize that all three are likely to exist in everyone in some degree or other. Dr. Rochlin spoke about the tyranny of technique, and Dr. Zetzel spoke about the intellectual framework into which one can place one's observations and thus hopefully gain some mastery over them. I think it is also important to think about these things particularly in relation to this potency problem.

There is an enormous feeling of impotence in the medical student, and often a similar feeling in the house officer, but perhaps it exists to a lesser degree in the older physician because he has lost those early dreams. He knows how limited he is, and he has given up those early fantasies that dog the student. It is very important to give a good theoretical framework within which one can strive for the mastery of the material. I think it is also very important that some techniques be put into the student's hands so that he does not feel so helpless. We see this strikingly in other branches of medicine. If a young medical student is assigned to the wards before he has any assurance regarding physical diagnosis, it is an upsetting experience for him, and it is helpful if he has something to do to master his anxiety. In this regard, there is one thing that both Dr. Zetzel and Dr. Kubie mentioned about which I feel strongly: it is extremely important that the student (medical student or resident) have a real feeling of activity. We need to let these students be active while providing them with an environment in which they can learn. We should drop the emphasis on what we teach them. I agree that we should pace our instructions, and that we should pay a good deal of attention to sequence, too, as Dr. Kubie mentioned. On the other hand, we should not get too frozen in sequence, for the young are often a lot smarter than we think they are; they often have a freshness, a sense of discovery, that is the greatest stimulus to their own learning. Moreover, it frequently is a stimulus to our own learning. For this reason, we should be humble when we decide upon what students should know. What we should try to do (and I think a number of people have said this already) is to tailor the course to the individual student. Again, I want to emphasize the need for the student to be active, for allowing him to learn by letting him make mistakes, because it is from our mistakes that we best learn.

DR. VALENSTEIN: Modes of therapy change as do the details of knowledge, but certain valid principles remain, even though they have to be modified to retain their validity. A meaningful appraisal depends primarily on a cumulative experience; after all, we have been applying psychoanalytic principles in the teaching of psychiatry for over 15 years. The outcome might have been anticipated, for Freud himself had misgivings about what might happen if analysis were to take root and become popular in America as in fact it has. What would be gained? What would be lost? Freud was afraid that psychoanalysis might lose from too much success.

Curiously, we are now concerned with exactly that possibility. We are quite willing to be relieved of the overestimation and overexpectations of psychoanalysis as a therapy, even of the overestimation of psychoanalytic psychotherapy, as a therapy based on psychoanalytic principles. What we would really regret losing is the psychoanalytic point of view with respect to human development and behavior, and with its pertinence to the teaching of medical students, physicians, and members of other professions dealing with human behavior. It would be an unfortunate paradox if we were to now pay the price of popularizing psychoanalysis by losing it as a scientifically valid, clinically useful body of knowledge and set of theories.

As the times changed, other approaches, such as small-group and family-milieu therapy, Pavlovian conditioning, and community social psychiatry have gained prominence. Fashions in therapy come and go as do the tides, and yet, if one only looks into the past, one will find the origin of what seems so novel. Through enlightened empiricism variations in the therapeutic approach may be developed to give added significance to the treatment of especially rigid or difficult patients. In this regard, though, psychoanalysis as a general psychology of human behavior can be particularly useful in evaluating innovations in therapy, and in explaining the success, or lack of success, the appropriateness or lack of appropriateness, of specific therapeutic modes for specific situations of illness.

This is highly relevant to the training of the psychiatrist, who often enters on his career with enormous enthusiasm. His therapeutic ambition may even encourage him to undertake a demanding interpersonal psychotherapy with an extremely sick individual, before whom a less expectant though more experienced psychiatrist might hesitate. This young resident may achieve a success with this very sick patient, which is explainable by his dedicated approach and compassionate interest in his patient rather than by his subtlety of insight. Psychoanalysis may provide an understanding of the course and outcome of treatment, even if it is not the most appropriate choice of therapy.

[134]

Dr. Rochlin has impelled me to put forth these queries: What is a psychoanalyst? What should be his role as teacher in the medical school and in the hospital? Should he leave behind his town garb as psychoanalyst and don the gown of medical academician? No, I don't think so. A psychoanalyst is not necessarily a person who practices analysis off the couch. He's a psychoanalyst by reason of his commitment to certain psychological points of view, and by his scientific perspective regarding human development and behavior, born of his training and of the historical evolution of psychoanalytic observations and theories.

These points of view are valid and applicable anywhere, and I am sure that Dr. Rochlin did not mean that they were not germane to teaching in the medical school and the hospital. He meant, I suppose, that the psychoanalyst should not enter the medical school and promptly proceed to make free-floating depth interpretations, as if he were in his analytic consulting room—and even there they should not be that free.

However, I do not suggest that there is some necessary antithesis in the two roles which I have come to regard as psychoanalytic "towners" and medical-school "gowners." We need not feel that those analysts who teach in psychiatric settings are analysts of a different breed from those who do not teach in the medical school or hospital but remain entirely involved with the independent institute or their individual practices. At the Beth Israel Hospital many of us have gained the feeling that a differentiation which suggests a mutual exclusiveness is incorrect. One can remain entirely in touch with psychoanalytic insights and understanding and yet be very flexible about how these are applied.

DR. KAHANA: There is much in the various discussions that

tempts me to pick up a number of issues, but I will have to make a choice. I appreciate Dr. Gitelson's remarks because he points up a problem in the use of models: they may freeze and thereby inhibit the resident's spontaneity as a clinician. This would be an unfortunate result. However, I do not believe that using models as a means of organizing observations and concepts must necessarily carry such a static connotation. When we try to comprehend new phenomena, one's thinking constantly vacillates between the specific and the general—which a model can represent. With respect to dedication: perhaps one's interest in other human beings and their problems can attain to a form of dedication. The psychotherapist must feel and convey some kind of physicianly or basically motherly dedication to the patient, if the latter is to enter into a therapeutic alliance.

I am in full accord with Dr. Zetzel's comments about the value of an objective framework of theory for the psychiatric resident, early in his training, to help him master the flood of provocative emotional material that confronts him in his patients. Of course, it is an individual matter. There are residents who are much better at finding their own way with a minimum of preconceptions. Others, right from the beginning, find a place for generalization and for conceptualization, not only to protect themselves but also as a means of organizing and assimilating their growing experience. Both the teaching of theory and the presentation of the general implications of specific cases can serve this purpose.

Dr. Kubie and I appear to be in agreement that much useful training centers around the knowledge of preconscious and conscious psychological material. This is often overlooked or not given sufficient emphasis.

DR. TARTAKOFF: In *The Aims of Education,* Alfred North Whitehead (1929) writes: "In a sense, knowledge shrinks as wisdom grows—for details are swallowed up in *principles.* The details of knowledge which are important will be picked up *ad hoc* in each avocation of life, but the habit of the active utilization of well-understood principles is the final possession wisdom" (p. 48).

For the past two decades, the category of resident psychiatrist has frequently overlapped that of candidacy in psychoanalytic training. In Boston, as in certain other centers, it has been the rule rather than the exception for psychoanalysts to teach candidates in training, not only in the Institute but also in the hospital. As a result, we find ourselves speaking a common language, sharing a common interest, and working within a common theoretical framework. Advantageous as this state of affairs may be from many points of view, it is not altogether without its hazards.

Dr. Rudolph Loewenstein is a training analyst of long standing, both in Paris and in New York, and a former president of the American Psychoanalytic Association. He parries the provocative question originally designated as the title of this symposium, "Can Dynamic Psychiatry Be Taught?" He offers an answer which goes far beyond the scope of this symposium, and yet also speaks directly to our subject.

DR. LOEWENSTEIN: I want to add two comments on psychoanalytic theory. I choose that topic advisedly, for it is a very narrow one. It does not cover all the problems encountered in teaching the interrelationship of analysis and psychiatry. Dr. Zetzel has expressed the view that today the young analyst who made the mistaken diagnosis might recognize the patient as a schizophrenic. This is very possible. But I doubt whether

[137]

our present knowledge of analysis is as adequate for predicting an outbreak of schizophrenia as it is for using analytic technique. Our theoretical knowledge serves us in understanding and analyzing our patients. In working with patients, an experienced clinician often uses his knowledge in an intuitive, more or less unconscious way. If we had the ability to translate this unconscious knowledge into theoretical terms, our theory would be very much richer.

I think the same is true for clinical psychiatry. I do not think there is (or need be) a dichotomy between clinical psychiatry and psychoanalysis. The fact is that the two bodies of knowledge do not overlap completely. A highly experienced clinician in psychiatry can observe certain things which as yet have not penetrated analytic theory. We might say that analytic theory has not yet learned enough from clinical observation. Dr. Gitelson is an exceptional man; he is an exceptional theoretician and an exceptional clinician. He is certainly one of the few people who could translate those innumerable clinical impressions—the implicit signs which he perceives—into psychoanalytic theory, and enrich it thereby. Psychoanalytic theory provides one of the best methods for teaching clinical observation, provided we understand that psychoanalytic theory does not have answers to all problems of the human mind.

DR. TARTAKOFF: Two years of residency, even under the most excellent conditions, prove to be too short a period in which to teach or treat residents and thereby impart wisdom and give the resident an opportunity to put it to the test. One important deterrent to inquiry on the part of the resident may be his fear of displaying his ignorance, a fear based on the ill-founded conviction that his teachers have all the answers.

Dr. Bond's point is well taken. Fortunately, there are some residents who feel free to develop their own technical style and maintain their own reservations regarding the immutability of established theory. Today, more than ever before, there are also residents who have the interest and special training in cognate fields which permit them to move in the direction of interdisciplinary cross-fertilization.

This symposium is addressing itself to one historic stage of a bridge-building endeavor, one in which the marriage of psychiatry and psychoanalysis has been consummated. It has as its aim the reevaluation of the offspring: *dynamic psychiatry* and a more general *medical psychology*. You have heard a wide range of comments on their present status and some predictions for their future. Even within the field of medicine, communication has been established and maintained with great effort. The bridges between dissimilar disciplines will be even more difficult to erect. It remains for the next generation to make significant strides in spanning the enormous distances between the natural sciences, the social sciences, and a general psychology of man.

PANEL III: PHYSICIANS IN THE COMMUNITY

Chairman, JOSEPH J. MICHAELS, M.D.

YESTERDAY MORNING, Dr. Tidd referred to Freud's paper of 1919, *On the Teaching of Psycho-Analysis in Universities.* I found it of considerable interest that when this paper was first published in a medical periodical in Hungary, the title was: "Should Psycho-Analysis Be Taught at the University?" In 1964, the question has been raised: "Can Psychiatry Be Taught?" Dr. Bibring presented us with an admirable examination of this important issue.

This morning we shall hear of the translations of psychoanalytic theory into their practical applications with a discussion of the complexities involved. Both papers deal with the experiences of psychoanalysts and pediatricians and may be considered paradigms for other physicians in the community.

"I Am Just a Pediatrician":
Educating Pediatricians in Dynamic Psychiatry

HENRY WERMER, M.D. and
MALVINA STOCK, M.D.

ALL OF US UNDERSTAND that many factors are involved in the
normal or deviant emotional and psychological growth of a
young child. One factor is the emotional climate in which a
child grows up. In this emotional climate there are certain
key figures which have a profound influence upon the small
ego and the great needs of the very young. First, there are the
parents and, to a lesser degree, the siblings. Second, in our
opinion, is the pediatrician or family physician. Third, and
appearing later, is the teacher. Here we will deal with the
second figure, the pediatrician, and describe our efforts to
enlarge, to vitalize, or revitalize the pediatrician's knowledge
of the psychoanalytic concepts of child development as he
may apply it to his patients.

Such education differs from teaching the basic concepts of
physiology, pathology, and the treatment of physical disorders, because it presents certain special problems. We refer

[143]

to the emotional reaction of the pediatrician that occurs in the course of this education and which presents an interference in his learning process. Later on in this paper we will elaborate on this important aspect.

In thinking about this presentation we recalled our activities as teachers of nonpsychiatric colleagues and students. This activity goes back many years. It began with schoolteachers in the Boston area. These educators, having had a prolonged and intensive contact with young children, were often the first to suspect an emotional disturbance in a child. Many of them also became aware that their own emotional reactions to a disturbed child often prevented them from acting in the most profitable manner. Simultaneously, however, they keenly felt the need for more knowledge of child development. The concern of teachers quickly turned into a request for education in dynamic psychology. A number of psychoanalysts, under the leadership of the late Dr. Leo Berman, responded with a program of seminars for educators, which is still being carried on.

Our experience in this program led to a lasting interest in finding ways of communicating psychological understanding to other nonpsychiatrists. Our orientation fitted neatly with the needs of a psychiatric service in a general hospital. When we joined the psychiatric service at the Beth Israel Hospital, we came into frequent contact with physicians in the medical and surgical departments who expressed an ever-increasing desire to understand their patients' personality structure and emotional needs. This desire also resulted in a request for a closer working relationship between psychiatry and all specialties of medicine. It was a natural development, therefore, that the psychiatrists became intimately involved—in addition to their treatment of patients—in teaching psychological

[144]

understanding to the nonpsychiatric staff. The appeal of the pediatricians led to a collaboration between Dr. Wermer and myself—of 14 years' duration—with the pediatric service and its staff, and both directly and indirectly with its patients.

Our work with the pediatric staff reflects the general philosophy of the psychiatric department, that is, to integrate into other branches of medicine a knowledge of dynamic psychiatry based on psychoanalytic concepts and theory. We deeply appreciate the role of Dr. Grete L. Bibring as our teacher and model. In our specific task we have been assisted by our associates, Drs. Meiss, Onesti, Selzer, and Stocking, and by Dr. Sherry, a psychiatrically trained pediatrician. We were encouraged in our undertaking by our teacher in child psychiatry, Dr. Lydia Dawes, as well as by the positive attitudes of the three successive pediatricians-in-chief, Drs. Gellis, Katz, and Berg.

Let us now share with you a recent experience. Some months ago we met with a group of pediatricians with whom we had worked regularly for several years. In previous seminars, we had been discussing interviewing methods and had illustrated such methods through verbatim reports of interviews by one of us in teaching fourth-year medical students. This prompted one of the pediatricians to volunteer his own interview, namely a diagnostic appraisal of a child and his family. The case itself was not unusual and constituted a routine part of the daily practice of a pediatrician. Such practice, in addition to physical problems, deals with developmental conflicts and crises, habit disturbances, and behavior disorders to which most children—at least in our culture—are prone. When the pediatrician presented his case history, other members of the group requested more detailed information. Even though the group appeared to be most congenial and harmonious, the doctor eventually replied to some of the questions in an almost despairing fashion, "I am just a pediatrician."

This spontaneous remark appears to be a most appropriate title for our paper. It illustrates an attitude of insecurity in regard to competence in matters of psychology which is quite common among our colleagues in pediatrics. Of course, there are a few who *a priori* reject medical-psychological concepts and cannot for example conceive that enuresis could be a phenomenon of emotional distress, a signal of disequilibrium within the child. Nevertheless, the vast majority of pediatricians with whom we have worked, whether they say so or not, are intensely interested in dynamic psychological factors.

As psychoanalysts we have always felt that pediatricians should have a firm grounding in the theory of psychological development. However, as indicated before, our whole program was initiated by the pediatricians' wish to learn more about psychological development and disturbances. In one instance a pediatrician approached us with a request for lectures and conferences, because he was concerned about a child who could not sleep. It was a young child, too young to become a subject for anything but a most superficial observational technique of interviewing. The fact that the child was suffering from separation anxiety became apparent only when the mother, in consultation with one of us, told us that she had spent several months at a local sanitarium where she had had shock treatment for a severe depression. During this period the child was cared for by the mother's aunt, who herself appeared to be suffering from chronic involutional melancholia.

Both the psychiatrist and the pediatrician were at first surprised by the fact that the child's doctor knew nothing about the mother's hospitalization. However, the mother explained this by saying, "After all, he is my pediatrician, and I did not want him to think badly of me." Please note that the mother did not say, "He is just a pediatrician." Quite to the contrary, she felt that this idealized man should not be burdened by knowing of her emotional illness and thereby think badly of her. She withheld her mental illness from the pediatrician but readily told the psychiatrist. She saw the pediatrician, rightly or wrongly, as being judgmental, and the psychiatrist as being able to hear the truth without turning his head. Obviously, she felt that a pediatrician and a psychiatrist have different value systems. Since there is already a paper on this topic, we will not discuss this issue except to state that we have given it constant attention. This attention to value systems is but one of the multiple approaches that have to be used in teaching our nonpsychiatric colleagues.

In our contacts with pediatricians, we have been impressed by the development of an increasing insecurity in regard to the psychological problems of children, an insecurity which seems to grow in direct proportion to the amount of time which separates the physician from the medical school and the hospital. The fact that, in contrast to his internship and residency, the pediatrician in his daily practice is exposed to an increasing number and scope of emotional problems enhances this feeling of insecurity. It seemed clear to us that we had to reintroduce the practicing pediatrician to some knowledge he had acquired earlier, in addition to offering some education in areas to which he had never been exposed during his medical school and residency training. It also became clear that reading the literature of Freud, Kanner, Spitz, Bettelheim, Mahler, and others obviously was not sufficient —it did not become integrated into the everyday thinking of the pediatrician.

In the course of our teaching a group of pediatricians, we repeatedly met with the experience, as mentioned earlier, that in spite of their adequate understanding of the material, they had a basic resistance to the concepts presented. Allow us to illustrate this resistance. In many seminars we discussed one of the cornerstones of analytic theory, namely, the theory of infantile sexuality, as postulated in Freud's "Three Essays on The Theory of Sexuality" (1905) and in other publications. The pediatricians reported their observations of infantile sexuality, of penis envy, of masturbation, and manifestations of oral and anal erotic drive. These topics came up by way of the clinical problems in pediatric practice, problems such as persistent thumb-sucking, soiling, or constipation, and the concern of parents over the sexual play of their children. Every pediatrician in the group was acquainted with the concept of the Oedipus complex and of castration anxiety.

In order to illustrate the variables of the oedipal conflict, we asked the group to read or reread Freud's classic paper on the analysis of a childhood phobia. We suggested this reading after we considered that the group had the capacity to truly comprehend the insights of this particular paper.

The evening this paper was discussed was a memorable one for two reasons. First of all, in reporting the paper, two pediatricians volunteered to take the roles of little Hans and his father. As they read the verbatim account of little Hans' "analysis," they played the role of father and son in an admirable fashion—evidence of their emotional involvement and intellectual comprehension of the material. From the lengthy discussion which ensued there emerged the second high point of the evening. A few of the pediatricians, perhaps induced by one whose desire for "scientific accuracy" was especially great, began to question the validity of little Hans' statements and thus the validity of Freud's interpretations. The argument was raised that little Hans was really an "innocent child," oblivious to sexual impulses and probably unaware of the difference between male and female. Further, it was inferred that Hans had been led to produce the remarkably clear material concerning his "widdler" by the "artificial, suggestive" comments made by his father.

To us as psychoanalysts, it became apparent that the group had acquired intellectual understanding, but the content of the case evoked a basic resistance. We drew a parallel from our daily analytic work, where we often find that an insight which the patient acquires and which we feel he has established as part of his self-knowledge, succumbs again to the power of resistance and the power of repression. We know that it may be dangerous to draw an analogy between the process of psychoanalysis and the imparting of conscious data in teaching. Nonetheless, we are convinced that the same basic resistance is in operation when the pediatrician knows yet doesn't know what he really knows. We could not attribute such a phenomenon to anything else, such as forgetting, lack of ability to comprehend, or even devotion to scientific accuracy.

Perhaps the statement "I'm just a pediatrician" reflects not only the pediatrician's uncertainty as to his knowledge about psychology, but also his emotional struggles in acquiring this knowledge. The intellectual acceptance, although helpful, in itself does not counteract the pediatrician's professional resistance based on his professional commitment and value system or his personal resistance rooted in his own unconscious. It thus became our task to find out whether or not the pediatrician can acquire the knowledge he needs, and if so, how we can help.

Psychoanalytic concepts deal with highly charged emotional material and tend to mobilize anxiety not only in the emotionally ill but in the emotionally healthy as well. The pediatrician often wards off this anxiety either by rejection, devaluation, or hostile argumentation. These defensive reactions handicap and block his learning processes and impair his effectiveness in understanding patients. This is why he withdraws behind "I'm just a pediatrician," which includes "I, too, am innocent and don't know of these things."

Our awareness of this problem led us to attempt to formulate our concepts in a way which would arouse the least anxiety; yet this did not fully explain how to make possible the true assimilation of those basic psychoanalytic concepts which would prove useful to him in his work. As stated before, it is clearly not enough to impart to the pediatrician our knowledge about psychic determinism and the power of the unconscious.

We try to orient the pediatrician to what we as analysts have derived from our own training, namely, that the present is determined not only by our environment but also very much by our past; that the future similarly will be determined not only by what we experience or can act up on now, but also by what happened to us years ago, and *above all, how we perceived these events.*

Our work as psychoanalysts frequently demands that we explore the depths of the unconscious. Thus we are reminded constantly by slips of the tongue, dreams, and preceptual distortions that psychic reality may determine behavior and symptomatology, and that this kind of reality may be *completely* divorced from actuality. We found that one of the most difficult tasks for the pediatrician is to recognize the meaning of psychic reality. This difficulty manifests itself

[150]

when he tries to assess a child's reactions. For example, we have often been asked why a child may remain so terrified of the minute discomfort of a throat examination or a vaccination, particularly when the pediatrician anticipates apprehension and gives reassurance. We could spend an entire morning discussing the basis for the child's terror of a stethoscope or tongueblade, and try to understand why he fearlessly climbs trees and cries for only a few seconds at the severe pain incurred by bumping his knee. An understanding of the child's reactions has to be "worked through" by using example upon example. Material we used in each conference or seminar included vignettes from clinical cases—from our personal experience, from the everyday practice of the pediatrician, and from our own children. In this way we illustrated an approach to the material, an attitude toward it based on deductions from observable data.

This method of sharing our knowledge also illustrates the principle on which our approach is based, namely, that it is not our intention to communicate this knowledge dogmatically as a body of revealed truths. It is rather to help the pediatrician to accept and assimilate these concepts intellectually and emotionally by mobilizing his curiosity, his interest, and his capacity to think through a certain phenomenon in the light of his experience—human and medical—and in the light of the psychological theories we uphold.

Similarly, too, we attempted to overcome the gap between the psychoanalyst's and the pediatrician's way of thinking about the patient's communications. The psychoanalyst almost automatically translates the patient's communications, play, behavior, and symptoms into the language of the unconscious, whether unconscious instinctual striving or unconscious defensive mechanism. To the pediatrician this is a most difficult undertaking and one which can be learned only very gradually. It must not, of course, be overlooked that skill in evaluating the unconscious requires a certain inner freedom, which exists to varying degrees in different individuals.

Let us now consider the techniques to be employed and the emotional relationship that has to exist between ourselves and the pediatricians. Although this relationship is difficult to describe we are convinced that it constitutes a *sine qua non* of a comfortable and productive learning process. In this relationship we psychiatrists are often the teachers, but frequently we are also the students. We believe that we have found, largely through our own training and experience, a correct emotional attitude on our part. Again, there is some similarity to the traditional concepts of psychotherapy and psychoanalysis. The analyst who feels superior to his patient or condescends to him is bound to fail. The psychiatrist who has anything but a genuine respect for his nonpsychiatric colleagues and, above all, for their humaneness, is bound to fail as an educator and even as a consultant. Mutual respect establishes a form of alliance which is the main vehicle for the learning process. Furthermore, certain features in this relationship bear resemblance to positive transference reactions and form a basis for the identification of the students with the instructor's attitude and approach to patients.

Our teaching techniques consist of the conferences mentioned before, as well as ward rounds and work in the outpatient clinic. They usually center on a discussion of an individual patient with his specific symptoms, conflicts, and personality structure. The case material is then used as a springboard for reviewing certain basic psychological concepts and neurotic syndromes, and oftentimes it offers the possibility of some prediction of a further development of the personality. Over the course of a number of years the subject of the psychological development of children has been given extensive consideration. Occasionally, the psychiatrist has functioned as an auxiliary to the pediatrician, either on the ward or in the outpatient department, by interviewing parents and by talking to children. In this way, the psychiatrist can demonstrate the technique of seemingly free-floating attention, which, however, is based on a firm grounding of normal and abnormal psychological development. In such joint interviews we have also been able to demonstrate to the pediatrician that it is not a lack of time but rather his own insecurity which handicaps him in eliciting data from the child and from the parents.

In the more or less didactic evening seminars, we have used material from a lecture by Anna Freud on "Psychoanalysis and Education" (1954). This paper is used as a model to illustrate the historical development of psychoanalytic theory from the time when it was largely a psychology of the id to the time when it included ego psychology.

Phases of libidinal development were discussed in detail and each theoretical presentation was illustrated by clinical examples that the pediatrician encounters in his everyday practice. It was possible to demonstrate the important function of the unconscious in the behavior of children, in symptom formation, and in character structure. We tried to illustrate how at times the inevitable conflicts of childhood, which are based on constitutional strivings of instinctual forces, can be alleviated and lead the child to mastery and further maturation. Also pointed out were the modes by which these conflicts may be diverted into psychopathology and fixation, thus leading to a crippling of the emotional life of the individual.

[153]

Considerable attention was placed on a theme attributed to Dr. Lauretta Bender that children have a natural drive toward healthy growth and development in spite of adverse circumstances. This aspect was emphasized because we were dealing not only with guilt-ridden parents but also with guilt-ridden doctors. Furthermore, it was necessary to stress that emotional conflicts are inevitable in spite of the best intentions of parents, physicians, and educators. In this context we discussed how early in the development of psychoanalysis it was thought that permissiveness in regard to the instinctual life of children could prevent the development of intrapsychic conflict; how parental experiments with extreme permissiveness ultimately backfired, making it apparent that the child needed the assistance of the parent to achieve control of his instinctual impulses if these were to be reconciled with the structure of his environment and our society in general. We pointed out that the development of a severe neurosis may occur when a child who is left to his own devices establishes much stricter controls than are necessary. We contrasted children reared in excessively permissive environments with those confronted by massive restrictive attitudes, and used these cases as an opportunity to discuss ego and superego development. A number of cases helped us to clarify "defensive mechanisms of the ego." As a sampling, let us mention a case of obsessional neurosis which gave us an opportunity to demonstrate reaction formation, isolation, and fixation in considerable detail. A case of anorexia nervosa in an adolescent girl made it possible for us to clarify the concept of the superego in dramatic detail; a case of an adolescent boy admitted to the pediatric ward who attempted suicide helped us to demonstrate the problem of feminine identification resulting in homosexual panic.

[154]

If our aims seem very ambitious, let us state that our intention was never to make psychiatrists or therapists out of pediatricians. We have actually been quite content with widening the scope of the pediatrician's point of view. We could sum up in a few sentences the goal of our work by stating that we have tried to give the pediatrician confidence in his capacity to differentiate between developmental phenomena and pathological fixation, that is, to differentiate between the normal crisis situations of childhood and the psychopathological states which lead to disabling neurosis or psychosis.

When is head-banging just playful head-banging or a more or less temporary release of aggressive tension, and when does it constitute a forerunner of a masochistic character attitude or a retreat into autistic oblivion? When is a food fad (one of the most common childhood disorders) simply a minor struggle within the child who wishes to express some antagonism or autonomy as would be acceptable at certain ages, and when does it become a snowballing problem of mother-child relationship, terminating for instance in obesity or anorexia nervosa? These are not easy questions, either for the psychiatrist or for the pediatrician. Let us keep in mind, above all, that the pediatrician is confronted with an ever-changing organism and that it is this month-to-month and year-to-year change of personality characteristics which is so befuddling. What adds to this difficulty is that the basic orientation of the pediatrician is often rooted in organic Virchovian pathology and the definite clear-cut physiological phenomena of Cannon, Selye, or the Corey cycle of sugar metabolism.

We have no way of assessing in a statistical manner the success or failure of our methods. Nor can we claim to be absolutely objective. We can only make certain guesses based on such factors as the kind of patients referred to our clinics by the pediatricians, and how this referral is handled with the family and with the clinic. These referrals and the innumerable consultations on the telephone, in the dining room of the hospital, or in the drugstore, give us clues as to the progress the pediatricians have made in becoming psychologically minded and truly knowledgeable. We stress "knowledgeable" because intuition cannot be taught, knowledge can. A further clue to the effectiveness of our efforts is the fact that we no longer see a rash of referrals by pediatricians who feel anxious and incompetent about handling a maturational crisis in a child's life. Nor do we have the impression any longer that the referral to a psychiatric children's clinic is a matter of last resort.

Some of the members of this panel are in the forefront of the movement which concerns itself with preventive psychiatry. Our work with pediatricians can be summarized as a small sector of this movement. Since the pediatricians are among the chief advisors to parents of young children, their orientation has an important influence on parental attitudes. They are, in a sense, practitioners of preventive psychiatry at the earliest stages of life. They must be conversant with such problem areas as when and how to wean, feeding schedules versus demand feeding, how to handle aggressiveness, toilet training, sibling rivalry, as well as the whole gamut of manifestations of infantile sexuality.

We hope that our imparting of psychological understanding to the pediatrician will result in a more comprehensive assessment and guidance of the child and the family. We have tried to help the pediatrician deal with the child's difficulty on a level which is neither too deep nor too superficial. For instance, we can expect that he will not talk about the castration complex to his patients nor will he ignore the fears deriving from it. We expect that he will be able to guide the parents of young children to find the happy-medium attitude toward the child's behavior, one which will be neither too permissive nor too controlling, but the correct middle-of-the-road attitude so essential for the growth of the child. Therefore, in our opinion, he will become a practitioner of comprehensive pediatrics and not see himself as "just a pediatrician."

DR. MICHAELS: Doctors Wermer and Stock stress the similarity of the therapeutic relationship between the patient and therapist and that between pediatrician and the psychiatrist. Thus they discuss an aspect of the therapeutic alliance, and I wonder whether we might say that what we require is a "professional alliance" when working with all kinds of colleagues. Their approach also utilizes a therapeutic attitude without carrying out psychotherapy. In all types of supervision and teaching, I think it is beneficial to have a therapeutic attitude, without undertaking psychotherapy. It is interesting to note how the attitudes that exist in this group correlate closely with some aspects of the teacher's attitude that Dr. Bibring discussed. When listening to people who work in groups, I am always impressed by the importance of group morale. Although we do not often speak about this factor (it may have a spiritual quality), it is really basic to learning and facilitates the identification of the student with the teacher.

Eight Pediatricians and a Child Psychiatrist: A Study in Collaboration

ALBERT J. SOLNIT, M.D.

MEDICAL EDUCATION AND PRACTICE represent a continuum in the quest for knowledge and in the refinement, translation, and application of this knowledge. In this report I shall focus on the description and assessment of a continuing effort to improve the translation and application of psychoanalytic medical psychology into pediatric education and practice. Some aspects of the historical background to this planned effort are contained in a 1954 report, "Teaching Comprehen-

This work has been supported in part by the Children's Bureau and National Institute of Mental Health, U. S. Department of Health, Education and Welfare; and the Connecticut State Department of Health. Their aid is gratefully acknowledged.

The author wishes to express his warm appreciation to his pediatric colleagues, who have demonstrated a capacity for scientific collaboration and professional camaraderie that is refreshing and inspiring. Although this study could not have been done without their unstinting cooperation and zest for inquiry, it is also true that the author must bear any responsibility for deficiencies or ambiguities in this report of our study.

[158]

EIGHT PEDIATRICIANS AND A CHILD PSYCHIATRIST

sive Pediatrics in an Outpatient Clinic" (Solnit and Senn, 1954). In that report, the American Academy of Pediatrics' definition of pediatrics is quoted in part as follows: "Pediatrics is that branch of the medical sciences which has to do with the factors influencing growth and development of individuals from birth to maturity" (p. 547). This 1954 report in part concludes:

1. Comprehensive medical care of the child is defined as the prevention and treatment of physical disease, and the supervision of healthy growth and development, physical and psychological. Through his comprehension of the physical, psychological and social forces that influence the child, the pediatrician enables the child and his family to take an active role in solving their health problems.

a. Every patient is an interesting person. It can be as satisfying and important to care for a 6-week-old infant who is well or a child who is going to camp, as for one who suffers from a rare disease.

b. The physician is faced with a patient (child) who is extremely dependent on parents or parental figures. The parents and child form a unit. It is the pediatrician's goal to help improve the health of the child by understanding the child's position in the unit.

2. The attitudes necessary for the practice of pediatrics are best acquired by the student through the demonstrations of his teachers and through his professional identification with them.

The next phase of our effort was initiated in 1957, when our senior pediatric residents, a group of pediatric practitioners who were part-time instructors, and a few of our full-time pediatric faculty met weekly to discuss the practical facets of psychological aspects of pediatrics. A child psychiatrist served as moderator as well as participant in this attempt to refine and apply psychological knowledge to the practice of pediatrics. The intentions and accomplishments of three years of these weekly seminars that developed around the case conference format can be summarized as follows:

Such a weekly exercise was expected to enable the practitioners who teach office pediatrics and the senior residents who would soon be confronted with the practical necessity of knowing the psychological aspects of pediatrics to learn from one another. The senior residents were within a year of entering either private practice or academic pediatrics, when they expected to devote a significant amount of time to teaching. We expected that this collaboration would tap a high level of motivation and provide this group of pediatricians with knowledge and techniques that would increase their versatility as practitioners and as teachers.

With rare exception, the practitioner group did not present their case material, although they participated fully in the discussions of cases presented by the pediatric residents. Case presentations were organized to provide a balanced spectrum from which to discuss the psychological aspects of pediatrics. These presentations led to discussions of all the developmental phases of childhood, a wide and practical range of psychological considerations in the practice of pediatrics, and selective follow-up discussions of certain patients and topics. The practitioners apparently preferred not to present their own case material. Several of them said that they did not have observations and historical data in depth compared to what a resident, in his more "leisurely" work, could gather for our seminar discussions. The practitioners appeared to be vaguely uncomfortable about presenting their case material to the pediatric resident members of our seminar.

Although a detailed discussion of the content of these Thursday seminars will be the subject for a separate report, it was agreed that it would be desirable to continue this study group. The child psychiatrist as moderator did not entirely agree, giving the impression that beyond the stimulation and involvement demonstrated during the conferences the practitioners had presented little evidence that the Thursday morning work had influenced their pediatric practice and teaching. At this time, the practitioners' contribution to the seminar was significant and was characterized by their focus on the realistic demands and opportunities of pediatric practice. These realities were formulated in the following terms: the erratic and harassing tempo and pace of practice; the patients' expectations of pediatricians; the large number of potential pathological problems for which the pediatrician was expected to be prepared, even though the problem turned up only rarely; the explosion of knowledge in the biochemical, genetic, and immunological sectors of pediatrics; and the demands that reflected the impact on pediatric practice of living in a rapidly changing and evolving urban society. The pediatricians often invoked these realities when translations and applications of psychoanalytic knowledge appeared to be wide of the mark as they were tested in the setting of the practitioner's everyday work.

Despite the paucity of material presented by the practicing pediatricians, it was clear that the pediatrician in practice could provide unique, cumulative, longitudinal observations and perspectives. It was also apparent that these data could

[161]

enrich and clarify our understanding of the course of neurotic difficulties, the vicissitudes of parental anxieties, and certain developmental characteristics and lags in childhood.

After a year of interruption the practitioners in the group suggested that we resume our Thursday seminars modified by the lessons learned in our collaborative work. For the past three years, eight of the practitioners have met with the child psychiatrist twice monthly for an hour and a half to continue our collaborative study of the psychological aspects of pediatrics. This time the child psychiatrist and one of the pediatricians became co-chairmen of the seminar. The eight practitioners were invited to participate on the basis of manifest interest and regional representation, especially because each of them was expected to enrich the teaching in our pediatrics department. The child psychiatrist, a psychoanalyst, aimed at a greater productivity in translating psychoanalytic formulations and hypotheses into pediatric knowledge, and in applying this knowledge to pediatric education and practice.

Other changes developed in our format. Each session was prepared in the following way. The child psychiatrist met with the pediatrician and his patient (child and family) who would then be the basis for our next conference. The interviews took place when practicable in the pediatrician's office; otherwise it was conducted in the child psychiatrist's office. The child and family were prepared for this meeting as a consultation in which a child psychiatrist and pediatrician would "put their heads together" in a collaborative effort to assist the child and his family in coping with a particular difficulty or set of difficulties. After this consultation with the patient and his family, which usually lasted an hour, the child psychiatrist and pediatrician met briefly to discuss immediate questions and offer advice that might be sensible and useful to the family. At this time the two physicians also compared observations and inferences which could be kept in mind for the study group. The next conference of the group was devoted to the discussion of this patient and became the basis for the seminar's consideration of the problems, questions, principles, and techniques that were most clearly suggested by the study and management of this patient. The recording of our experiences was two-fold: the pediatrician prepared a two- to three-page case report before the conference; in addition, an expert secretary, who had also recorded many of the 1957-1960 meetings, kept running shorthand notes of the seminar, which were immediately transcribed into a typed draft for the child psychiatrist, upon termination of the conference.

So much for an outline of our history and mode of functioning. Perhaps we can enliven the outline by briefly describing the members of this seminar. The child psychiatrist-psychoanalyst member of the group, trained originally in pediatrics, has been engaged in teaching the psychological aspects of pediatrics for many years. All the practicing pediatricians are valued as excellent clinical teachers in the Department of Pediatrics. They usually took the same chairs at the conference table. The rest of the group was comprised of the following physicians.

Dr. Steady has been practicing solo for more than five years in a northern suburb of New Haven. He is a patient, thoughtful person who recently was elected to the Board of Education in his small town.

Dr. Judge has been practicing solo for more than five years in a neighboring community. He is cautious, reflective, and involved in a number of the community organizations for which his interests and training have qualified him, including the Board of Health of his community, and a children's institution. He is an afficionado of orchid culture.

Dr. Gentle is practicing in partnership with a colleague in New Haven who shares with him a passionate interest in social and psychological aspects of child development. He is an expert in pediatric cardiology and the chief pediatrician of an agency devoted to the rehabilitation of handicapped children. Dr. Gentle is a devoted and leading member of a local chorale group.

Dr. Yankee, who has practiced solo in New Haven for more than 15 years, is highly respected for his thoughtfulness. He is active in the affairs of the local medical society, and is perhaps the most gifted teacher of medical students in the group. Dr. Yankee is a sailing enthusiast.

Dr. Eager has practiced in partnership with Dr. Grapple in a nearby town for about five years. Dr. Eager is involved in many community activities and is under great pressure to keep up with his growing practice.

Dr. Grapple forsook a promising career in research to enter private practice five years ago in partnership with Dr. Eager. For several years, Dr. Grapple was able to continue his research interests on a part-time basis while in practice.

Dr. Perspective has been practicing in partnership for more than 15 years in a town over 30 miles from New Haven. His persistent interest in what the pediatrician can do to prevent psychological difficulties has had a formative influence on our collaborative efforts. Dr. Perspective is president of a state pediatric society.

Dr. Fellowship has practiced solo for 10 years, having prepared himself by special training with Dr. Edith Jackson. He is involved in a number of community activities, including a child-guidance clinic, a settlement house in New Haven's Negro ghetto. At present Dr. Fellowship is president of the New Haven Area Mental Health Association.

This seminar is heavily weighted by devoted pediatric practitioners who are deeply involved in teaching and in applying their knowledge and experience for the benefit of the communities in which they live with their own families. All of them are under 50 and over 30—the modal age being about forty.

What has this unusual group learned, taught, and demonstrated? The answers to these questions have been formulated by the child psychiatrist and discussed with the study group. Before proceeding to the answers, it will be appropriate to state an underlying assumption involved in our collaboration, specifically, that the primary and secondary prevention of psychological disorders and deviations cannot and should not be regarded as being strictly within the province of child psychiatry. Child psychiatry has the task of adding to the basic knowledge of child development and of training child psychiatrists. This responsibility includes the uncovering of new knowledge, and the refinement, translation, and distribution of this knowledge of child psychiatry to those who are responsible for child care and child health, especially parents, educators, and physicians.

The results of this three-year collaboration will be outlined from three points of view. The first is the impact of this work on the individual pediatrician's teaching of medical students, especially the seniors in our outpatient pediatric clinic; second, the impact of the collaborative exercise on the private practice of each of the pediatricians; and third, a description of the sectors of psychoanalytic knowledge that were translated and the degree to which these translations appeared to become useful pediatric knowledge.

In regard to the impact on teaching, three observers inde-

[165]

pendently rated each of the pediatricians. These observers
were a pediatrician, a social worker, and the child psychiatrist, all of whom have been intimately involved in teaching
clinical pediatrics to senior medical students for many years.
There was an impressive consensus in this evaluation. Three
of the eight pediatricians were considered to have become
outstanding teachers, to a significant degree in association
with the collaborative study of psychological aspects of pediatric practice. Two of the pediatricians were difficult to evaluate as teachers because their major teaching involvements
are in specialty clinics, where they are valued for their interest and dependability. Three are considered to have been
sound teachers whose quality of teaching was unchanged in
association with their involvement in this collaborative exercise. One of this group has recently become active in our
teaching program for senior medical students, and there is
some evidence that he may become one of the outstanding
teachers. There was also an agreement by the evaluators that
none of the eight pediatricians has become less effective or
less clear in his teaching during these three years.

The impact of the collaborative exercise on the private
practice of each pediatrician has been evaluated subjectively
by each of the participants. The consensus was that it had enabled them to work more realistically with a small number of
patients having complicated psychological problems. However, they felt that the greatest impact of our collaborative
experience had been to advance their effectiveness and satisfaction in the anticipatory care of the majority of their
patients. There was a striking agreement as to their reactions
to patients with psychological problems. Instead of feeling
harassed and eager to refer such patients to some other physician or special clinic, the physician's interest in such patients

[166]

was associated with his knowing that there was a forum in which he could discuss the particular patient. Part of this expectation was determined by his awareness that there was a collaborator available to assist in the assessment and planning for this patient. Each of the pediatricians in his own way also alluded to a greater comfort in his everyday work and to an increased sensitivity to his patients' psychological characteristics and difficulties.

In studying and treating psychological problems in childhood, the pediatricians demonstrated what analysts have learned over the years: it is important to have a group with whom one can discuss his experiences as he gradually arrives at an understanding of his patients and through which one may assess the therapeutic effectiveness of understanding put into action.

The past history of this collaborative group may contribute to this assessment of their clinical pediatric work. Through work in the Yale Department of Pediatrics and in the local and state pediatric societies, they have all known one another for many years. They all share a deep admiration for Dr. Milton J. E. Senn, Director of the Child Study Center until 1966 and Chairman of the Yale Department of Pediatrics from 1951 to 1964, who has both directly and indirectly influenced their professional development. Also, all eight had had their pediatric training in part or completely at the Yale Medical Center; four of them had graduated from the Yale School of Medicine before receiving all or part of their pediatric training in New Haven. Thus we can view the three years of collaboration as an extension and elaboration of the postgraduate studies that are so necessary for the modern physician. Although each physician bears the responsibility for his continuing medical education (Spink, 1964), professional isolation carries a significant risk for most physicians. Isolation in solo clinical work is probably one of the most important reasons why many pediatricians become bitter and feel helpless about the realities of their practice.

Our clinical studies and discussions covered a wide range of common psychological and developmental difficulties. Although the content and findings of these studies cannot be described completely or discussed in detail in this presentation, it will be pertinent to outline some of the psychoanalytic views and formulations that were useful in our discussions. These applications of psychoanalytic knowledge to pediatric practice were examined for their usefulness and their limitations.

There were four sectors of psychoanalytic theory that were repeatedly applied in our collaborative work. First, the dynamic and genetic aspects of developmental tasks and patterns of object relationships in a family setting came up repeatedly in the context of understanding individual patients and their difficulties. For example, the discussions of a child's reactions to death in a family required us to examine the developmental tasks confronting that child at the time, as well as the family constellation and modes of personal relationships in the family. Such discussions elaborated into the consideration of developing object relationships, including various oedipal constellations, and the influence of object-loss and mourning reactions on ego development. The considerations in this area also included other aspects of ego psychology, particularly the changing meaning and influence of object representations, the developing sense of time, and the impact of the adaptive and maladaptive functions of memory on the child's unfolding capacities. Developmental tasks became the conceptual frame for presenting these psychoanalytic insights.

The theory of trauma and fixation, an overlapping sector of psychoanalytic knowledge, also was essential for our collaborative work. This came up repeatedly and characteristically in the context of child-rearing practices that magnified the problems of the children we were evaluating. For example, a five-year-old boy was repeatedly punished (traumatized) in an effort to compel him to stop soiling. Spankings had been a repeated disciplinary device to promote "character building." In another instance a boy of three and a half had marked fears of going to sleep at night. It became clear that these fears had become intensified and elaborated in a setting in which the child was regularly taken into the parental bed. It could be demonstrated that this child's castration anxiety and sleep disturbance had been magnified and elaborated by the traumatic overstimulation to which he was repeatedly subjected.

A third sector of psychoanalytic theory—as to what constitutes mental health (Hartmann, 1939a; A. Freud, 1959)—contributed to pediatric assessments of psychological health. These assessments included an inventory of the patient's assets as well as of the liabilities of symptoms and developmental deviations. The pediatricians had an unusual, perhaps an untapped, reservoir of knowledge about their patients which had been cumulative, often from birth. This longitudinal perspective enabled the child's physician to know about capacities that were developing and resources that were adaptive despite a physical or psychological difficulty. For example, the psychoanalytic theory of autonomous ego functions (Hartmann, 1939b) was formulated as a result of

the study of an eight-year-old girl with school-learning difficulties. This enabled the pediatrician to advise remedial
assistance to the child for her underachievement, as well as
adequate opportunities for her to exercise and elaborate capacities that had not been invaded by a troubled identification with her tempestuous father.

The fourth sector of psychoanalytic theory that was
applied was a translation of the concept of partial identifications in the service of the child's alliance with his pediatrician. Discussions, especially of younger children, regularly
included the ways in which the pediatrician could help the
patient to relate to him in a manner that would allow the
child to identify in part with the physician. Taking over certain of the doctor's attitudes toward the child and his health
problems enabled the latter to gain a clearer recognition of
his condition at the same time that it mobilized his interest
and energies to overcome his illness. For example, through
the use of a few toys (a ball, crayons and paper, and a flash-
light), the pediatrician created a pleasant and appropriate
atmosphere in which to talk to a boy of five and a half who
was afflicted with enuresis. Through an identification with
the pediatrician, the child was encouraged to discuss the bed-
wetting with his doctor, and was consequently able to
strengthen his own effective determination to overcome this
"babyish habit."

There were many other psychoanalytic propositions that
became useful to the pediatric armamentarium. These
emerged as discussions of the pleasure and reality principles,
the unconscious motivations of parents, the levels of stimulation and experience that are appropriate to children at different stages of their development, and various derivatives of

psychosexual and psychoaggressive development that were observed in our patients.

* * *

At the beginning of the three years, there were a number of different clinical problems presented as the basis for our discussion. These included families in which either a child or parent had died suddenly; a six-year-old boy with a school-learning problem; a five-year-old boy with fecal retention; a 10-year-old boy with enuresis and extreme passivity; and a large variety of behavior problems and anxiety reactions in children under the age of 14 (see Table 1). After about six months, the seminar group gradually became aware that one of the main continuing themes of our seminars was that of parents who were less concerned and less willing to take action about the symptoms and developmental deviations of their respective children than was the responsible pediatrician. This led to an intense, at times heated, exposition of the liabilities and offensive qualities of parents who were not cooperating with the pediatrician in his efforts to protect the child's health and to guide parents and child.

In many previous discussions there had been explicit elaborations of how to recognize the universal tendency of pediatricians to compete with parents or to view parents as those against whom children should be protected. A further consideration of why these patients had been selected by the pediatricians for a collaborative study with the child psychiatrist indicated that these parents were among the most trying people with whom pediatricians work. It was observed that there was a tendency for pediatricians to moralize about the psychological difficulties in such families, and that there was little satisfaction in trying to be of assistance to their children. This tendency was exposed in our discussions by contrasting the pediatrician's questioning attitudes toward a patient with an infectious disease and his attitudes toward a patient whose parents appear to ignore a developmental or psychological disorder. In the former, his attitudes could be paraphrased by the question, "How did this come about and what are the influences, chemical and environmental, that will enable the child to overcome the infection?" Concerning the psychological disorders in these families his attitudes often were represented first by the question, "Who should be blamed for the child's plight?" Often the pediatrician unrealistically implied that, if he could not find someone to blame for the child's difficulties, he would have to blame himself.

Having identified the vexing theme of the parent who appears uncooperative, the collaborative group moved toward a changed perspective of studying individual children in such families with the goal of understanding rather than of changing the parents and child. After minimizing the pediatrician's demand that the parents change significantly, it was possible to use further psychological understanding of such families as an aid to establishing an avenue through which a doctor-parent alliance could be established. This enabled our group to become more deliberate in studying how to work toward a referral for psychiatric evaluation and treatment when it was clearly indicated. Actually, one out of 10 of the patients we studied was referred to a child psychiatric clinic.

There were many other facets of this collaborative study that will be described in other reports. As this study and others (e.g., that of Leonard Weiner, Boston University, personal communication) indicate, the question "Can psychiatry be taught?" can be answered in the affirmative. This report suggests that the next questions to consider concern what psychoanalytic knowledge should be translated and applied in pediatric practice and education, and how to accomplish this most effectively. This study in collaboration is one approach to the answer of such questions.

TABLE 1

PSYCHOLOGICAL ASPECTS OF PEDIATRICS
COLLABORATIVE CONFERENCE TOPICS 1961-1964

Date	Name	Age	Diagnosis or Presenting Complaints
9-14-61	Abigail	5	Death of sibling from malignancy
9-28-61	Bonny	6-½	Sudden accidental death of mother; patient was also in an accident
10-12-61	Ralph	6	School-learning problem
10-26-61	Paul	5	School-learning problem
11-9-61	Stanley	10	Enuresis and school-learning problem
	Follow-up on Bonny		
11-21-61	Follow-up discussions		
12-21-61	Samuel		Constant rocker; sleep disturbance; behavior problem
1-4-62	Daniel	3	Bowel and bladder control; sexual education
1-18-62	Alvin	3-½	Sleep problem
2-1-62	Felicia	2-⅔	Constipation
2-15-62	Basil	6	Adopted child, impulsive autistic behavior: lying and stealing
2-29-62	Michael	3	Parents killed in air crash
3-29-62	Morton	9	Stealing and hiding mother's underwear
4-12-62	Anticipatory guidance in adolescence		
4-27-62	Thad	12	Separation anxiety
5-24-62	Follow-up discussions		
6-15-62			
9-27-62	Adolescents as a group	12 to 18	Developmental tasks in adolescence
10-11-62	Laurie	11	Jittery and feels nauseated in school
10-25-62	Robert	11	Enuresis

TABLE 1 (*continued*)

11-7-62			
12-13-62	Evan	10	Facial tics
12-20-62	Charles	9	Encopresis
1-3-63	Eugene	7	Enuresis
1-13-63	Neil	6 wks.	Parents' reaction to birth of defective child
1-31-63	Evan's follow-up		
2-7-63	Theresa	6	Enuresis
2-21-63	Diana	7	Compulsive masturbation
2-28-63	Raymond	5	Wild behavior and school-learning difficulties
3-14-63	Augusta	3-½	Sleep disturbance after infant brother died by strangulation (strap of toy)
3-28-63	William	11	Enuresis
4-11-63	Rachel	3-½	"Couldn't have bowel movement on toilet"
5-9-63	Elias	5-½	Enuresis
5-16-63	Nancy	5-½	Encopresis
5-21-63	Dennis	5	Wild behavior
5-23-63	Dirk	6-½	School underachievement and effeminate behavior
10-17-63 & 10-24-63	Kathy	8	Sleep disturbance and fearful behavior
10-31-63	Richard	10	Headaches and abdominal pains
11-14-63	Elsie	10	Phobic reactions
12-12-63	Leonard	5	Stool retention
12-21-63 & 1-2-64	Frank	11	Encopresis
1-23-64	John	12	Chest and abdominal pains; poor impulse control
2-6-64	Curtis	15	Acute depression; poor school work; repeated upper respiratory infections
2-20-64	Mary	5-½	Negativistic behavior
3-5-64	Axel	5	Teasing; discipline problem
3-26-64	Alice	7-½	Encopresis and enuresis
4-16-64 } 4-22-64	Discussion with Dr. Anna Freud		
5-14-64	Discussion of plans for 1964-65		
6-3-64	Denise	8	School-learning difficulties and rebellious behavior
6-18-64	Larry	4-½	Encopresis

[174]

Discussion

DR. MICHAELS: Dr. Loewenstein has stated that a psychiatrist performs an implicit translation from the general and abstract to the individual and concrete. Doctors Stock and Solnit have admirably shown us just how this can be done. It is interesting to note that the psychiatrists who presented these papers are both training analysts. They have used their analytic training and experience; they have applied their ideas in different settings and still have maintained their professional identities as psychoanalysts.

DR. EWALT: There is a story of a man who visited his son at college. He went to an economics class with his son on the day that they were having a quiz. At the end of the hour the man approached the instructor and said, "I went to school here about 30 years ago. These questions look similar to those I had on a quiz when I was here." The instructor replied, "Oh, indeed, they are exactly the same questions. The answers have changed from year to year."

When I read these papers (and they are excellent), I wondered why we talk about these issues today, in the fall of 1964.

Drs. Jack R. Ewalt, George E. Gardner, M. Ralph Kaufman, and Erich Lindemann delivered prepared discussions by invitation.

Drs. John P. Spiegel, Silvio J. Onesti, Jr., and Henry Wermer took part in the general discussion.

[175]

Thirty years ago, when I started my residency at the Colorado Psychopathic Hospital, Dr. Edward Gregory Billings had just come to Colorado from Johns Hopkins to start what was then called the psychiatric liaison department. He was going to integrate psychiatry with medicine, surgery, pediatrics, etc. We discussed precisely these issues in one of the first seminars I attended as a psychiatric resident. Thirteen years ago, when I came to Boston, Dr. Leo Berman and Dr. Ed Landy already had a clan of "Bermanites" in the Newton school system who were devoted to applying the practical aspect of analytic ego psychology to teaching children. So my first reaction to our current enterprise was, "My God, are we this far behind the times at Harvard that we are having a symposium like this?" Then I thought, "No, that's not right. If we are still discussing it, it's because we haven't solved the problem." Some clues as to why we are still discussing it 30 years later (I think we may be doing the same thing 30 years from now) are contained in both of the papers. Each of the problems they point out are problems inherent in the process of trying to communicate psychoanalytic insights—or psychiatric insights in general—to people accustomed to dancing to a different tune, or at least to one written in a different key. They point out, and probably correctly, that part of this problem is resistance, the resistance of the sort encountered in analytic therapy. If this is discouraging, it is because we are aware of the difficulties involved in analyzing resistance even when the patient is on the couch under voluntary scrutiny. Consider how much more versatile and elusive resistance is when manifested by our colleagues in clinical and educational settings. The defenses used, for example, by members of the curriculum committee vary from denial and rejection to what I consider much more malignant: reaction formation, characterized by apparently

[176]

wholehearted acceptance and application of analytic insights. However, that application is carried to the point of absurdity, resulting in ultimately damaging effects upon the meaningful use of analytic knowledge and skill.

While the problem of communication of meaningful information has been encountered in both studies, both have found that long-term work with a small group of pediatricians met with notable success. We may have to make such education generally available—particularly to most (if not all) pediatricians—if they are to discharge fully their responsibilities as a major resource in the promotion of mental health and the prevention of mental disease. We know how to handle personal resistance, but it requires long and expensive treatment, and treatment to which most of our colleagues would not submit. Insofar as personal resistance is concerned, most psychoanalysts know that any of us sees in a given situation only that which he considers of significance or importance, and nothing more. People of different educational backgrounds and experience will see and hear markedly different aspects of any given situation. Furthermore, their interpretations of the significance of the events as they see and hear them will vary with their own information and experience. Consider a glass of beer. The chemist would see its physical properties: wet (in America cold, in England warm), brown, liquid. To our "chemical colleagues," it is made up of sugar, water, alcohol, and the most delightful part of it (known as congenors), which accounts for the flavor and is bad for the liver. To college and medical students, beer is for releasing tension. To a Baptist minister in the Bible Belt of Texas, it is a threat to man's morality. In short, everyone interprets it in terms of his own life experience and knowledge.

If the pediatrician is to acquire a useful set of analytic concepts, he must incorporate such knowledge into his education so that, when he begins to deal with the more advanced clinical concepts, he has an easily available frame of reference. How early is it appropriate? I think probably in college, certainly not later than the very first year of medical school. Doctors Wermer and Stock have pointed out that the more recent medical-school graduates grasp these concepts the more easily. This fact is borne out by two more objective studies. One, done in New Jersey some years ago, has shown that recent medical-school graduates were able to obtain a better grasp of, and profited more easily from, graduate education in psychiatric concepts than those who had been out of school for some time. In our own Joint Commission survey sample of ordinary people's opinions, we have found that the younger and better educated persons tend to conceive of their troubles, problems, and tensions in psychological terms, while the older ones tend to view their problems in terms of physical disorders (e.g. stomach or heart trouble). Although these studies are not always comparable, they all point in the same direction. If we wish to achieve meaningful results with these people, we must begin to work with them early in their careers. Other educators maintain that an intellectual grasp of analytic theory and principle will automatically carry over to insight and knowledge in the clinical setting. However, if as part of his general association pattern a doctor is accustomed to looking at all situations in terms of analytic concepts, it may well be that he will, under proper instruction, learn to apply his knowledge more quickly to clinical and family situations.

It may be redundant, but I would like to call attention to the problem of overgeneralizing from a little bit of knowledge. We can avoid the pitfalls and absurdities if we remind ourselves and our colleagues, when working with techniques

[178]

to ameliorate stress, that a stress is in the mind of the person under stress. What is stressful to one person may not be stressful to another at all. My colleagues sometimes poke fun at me for my devotion to sports-car races—my favorite form of relaxation. (Once I was taking Dr. Malamud to catch an airplane, and we missed it. So we drove to the neighboring town and caught it there. Bill has since impugned my reputation, in a semiserious way, all over the world.) However, I know people who go fishing for relaxation and I can think of no greater form of stress than to be tied to the end of a fishpole, waiting for some stupid fish to grab hold of the bait.

In teaching our colleagues about things that are stressful, we must remember that stress is a highly individualized feeling, and that one cannot make general statements, based on theory, about what will be stressful for John Jones in contrast to Mary Smith. We must not expect the patient to conform to our concepts of stress, but rather encourage him to cope with what he sees in relation to his own experience. We must take steps to avoid having inadequate knowledge lead to overgeneralization. If we go beating about the bushes in the mental-health field, we must have the support of our colleagues, but in turn our colleagues must be informed and adequately prepared to use the information.

Dr. MICHAELS: Dr. Ewalt suggests that we should not pay as much attention as we do to the problem of resistance. However, I believe that there are four aspects of resistance that are becoming clearer and more suitable for examination, such as the two that Dr. Ewalt mentioned: the professional-medical type of resistance, and that of the individual confronted with an emotional problem. A third aspect concerns the values that Dr. Bibring mentioned last night—the difference between the inclusive-exclusive points of view of the psychiatrist versus those of the physician, the organic point of view versus the holistic point of view—while the fourth involves the use of the realistic situation as a resistance. All these physicians are so busy, have too many patients and too little time.

DR. GARDNER: Four of the six basic questions usually assumed to be of paramount importance in respect to any educational task, experiment, or enrichment have been answered with clarity and comprehensiveness by our distinguished panelists. In their outlines of the problems involved in the teaching of dynamic or psychoanalytic psychiatry to pediatricians, they have dealt with the aims, the desired content, the various methods of teaching this body of knowledge, and the experience and educational background of the student we are trying to teach. In short, they have given us answers of great importance and inclusiveness to the question put by Herbert Spencer's (1884) book, *What Knowledge Is of Most Worth?*
However, there are two additional significant questions in teaching new knowledge and skills to any student of any age. (In respect to these fifth and sixth questions, one must bear in mind that acquiring new knowledge demands a more or less drastic modification of the old familiar knowledge and skills.) The fifth question (and problem): What is the student's "mind-set" or motivation (essentially his identity) in his attempt to acquire the new knowledge? The sixth (closely allied to the fifth) is: Does the student have realistic expectations of what he may gain from this new knowledge and what satisfactions can be derived from his new learning or skills in substitution for the old? Both questions are of great significance in teaching psychoanalytic concepts to pediatricians.
Let us now turn for a moment to pictorial thinking. In the

British Museum there hangs a famous canvas, "The Doctor," by one of Britain's moderately distinguished painters, Sir Luke Fildes (1844-1927). This picture of the doctor at the bedside of an acutely ill child, with the trustful and hopeful parents in the background, is well known to all of you. In reference to our fifth problem, this picture illustrates better than any thousands of words the unconscious, and possibly the conscious, fantasy the pediatrician has of his role. The picture shows the bases for his motivation to learn, the goal he expects to reach, and the satisfactions he expects to have. Through his knowledge, he will become the conqueror of pain and the man who can restore health and happiness to this child and his family.

Unfortunately, in our present day society, Sir Luke's canvas is no longer a fantasy based on reality. The last half-century has brought a succession of preventive and curative waves of vaccines, sera, antibiotics, and chemotherapeutic agents. With this change comes the painful necessity of changing much of the above fantasy—a fantasy which is basic to the pediatrician's motivation and basic to his identity and professional satisfactions. However, professional nostalgia is difficult to eradicate and, like individual and social nostalgias, it does affect, sometimes destructively, the motivation to learn, to progress, and to assume newer although possibly equally satisfying roles.

But there is an additional feeling in Sir Luke's picture that never escapes my attention, the feeling of anxiety. On the faces of the child's parents, anxiety is obvious. These anxieties about pain and about the child's life or death come through more strongly because of the calm denial painted on the face of the physician. But anyone looking at the picture feels other anxieties in addition to the central one of life or death. When

[181]

awake, the child feels anxieties about his unfulfilled needs for comfort, for mobility, for future action, for future play, and future fun. There is also anxiety connected with what this child may mean to each parent, to his siblings, to his whole family. And finally, there is my anxiety (and theirs, including the doctor's) about the kind of child this patient will be when he recovers from his crisis. What will this mean in respect to his future physical and mental development?

Therefore, one segment of the fantasy of the pediatrician's future identification (as the educated instrument which can, in a crisis, alleviate pain, eradicate disease, and sustain life) must be drastically modified. Fantasy about his professional role can and should take place. In modifying his role, he is required, simultaneously and automatically, to seek new kinds of anticipated satisfactions in his professional role. He must substitute something for the fantasy of himself being the savior who alleviates pain and suffering and prevents death. This is the sixth problem in teaching.

The remaining contents of the fantasy picture could and should afford both strong motivations and great satisfactions for the pediatrician, were he to realize its ubiquitousness, its meaning, and its real toll. He will be in a position to realize the opportunity only if we as psychoanalysts create within him (by our training) a heightened sensitivity to it. I refer specifically to the problem of anxiety, the anxiety present in children and in parents, the anxiety that is so significant an element in child-parent relationships, not only in crises and times of stress, but in all processes of infant and child development, both for the child and for the parent.

This leads us directly to the question of content in teaching psychoanalytic and dynamic psychiatry to the pediatrician. One of the most important areas of our increasing body of psychoanalytic knowledge is the one that deals with the sources, the expressions, the displacements, and the meanings of anxiety in both children and adults. Our literature abounds with evidence supporting the fact that anxiety is the main disabling factor in the neuroses, the behavioral disabilities, and in all the maturational arrests and regressive maneuvers in childhood development, in personality, and in learning.

Although I subscribe completely and enthusiastically to the suggestions for educational content mentioned by both our principal speakers, I feel that the pressure and potency of anxiety—as the equivalent of pain and suffering and as a response to actual or fantasied mutilation or death—should be stressed in every teaching exercise, and that our published works on this subject should be emphasized in our prescribed reading lists.

A thorough appreciation of anxiety and of its expressions is of particular significance to the pediatrician because he deals with both children and parents. For anxiety is generated not only in times of crises (in sickness, in death, in separation) but is a reactivated force (however slight) whenever an infant or child makes any significant advance in its education and training. In his evaluation of a developmental step required and taken, or one not taken, or one shortly to be taken, it is necessary for the pediatrician to know that anxiety—what I would term "developmental anxiety"—will supervene, at least transiently, and that this developmental anxiety which is active in the child at the time a growth process emerges is also present in the parent. The pediatrician will receive a true sense of satisfaction from realizing that he has the diagnostic skill to understand anxiety as well as the clinical skill to modify it, and that by so doing can help prevent the transformation of developmental anxiety into disabling anxiety.

[183]

In all my teaching of pediatricians, along with my colleagues, I have stressed the overriding importance of knowing the developmental stages in child personality development and in child mental processes (or ego development).
I have also stressed the importance of the impact of crises and
the continuity of the child-parent emotional climate in helping the child find a successful solution to his developmental
tasks. However, from my own observations and from the reports of my two colleagues, it seems clear to me that the pediatrician needs more than an intellectually built-in "Psychoanalytic Gesell Scale." For the sake of his own motivation to
alleviate suffering and because such knowledge is central to
his job, the pediatrician must be made aware of anxiety and
must realize that, if he learns to treat anxiety expertly, he can
again assume his traditional role of one who detects, prevents,
or alleviates this equivalent of present pain, this harbinger
of possible future severe disability. In this way, the peripheral
areas of Sir Luke Fildes' picture enter the center of our
vision.

As an extension of my main thesis, I would like to comment
on a significant developmental stage now being reached by
two professions closely allied to us—pediatrics and child psychiatry. Both these medical specialties are relatively young.
Both have been called on in their infancy and youth to take a
leap in professional development that will fulfill a recognized
community health need: a comprehensive child-care program
for their patients. At the same time, each is required to continue giving adequate care and treatment to extremely ill
(physically or psychologically) children. Here, indeed, is a
source of "developmental anxiety" that one can detect in a
growing organism when changes are demanded. I think I can
detect my developmental anxiety in the titles selected for this

[184]

section of our symposium: "I Am Just a Pediatrician," and "Eight Pediatricians and a Child Psychiatrist." I have faith that this developmental anxiety will not become disabling anxiety.

Because I have used this British painting to structure my remarks and have commented on the possible power of unconscious fantasies and identifications, I cannot resist a final comment on Sir Luke. As a psychoanalyst, it is of interest to me (and I hope to you) to know that this artist—whose world-renowned painting, "The Doctor," was the favorite picture of Queen Victoria and resulted in his knighthood—was christened in infancy in honor of St. Luke the physician!

DR. KAUFMAN: I should like to thank Doctor Michaels for his introduction, and to congratulate Doctor Bibring and her staff on the excellent department at the Beth Israel Hospital. I have a certain paternal pride in the department, since, as most of you know, I was asked to reorganize it in 1933 and was extremely fortunate to have Dr. Bibring as a member of my staff, so that when I entered the service in 1942, she was in a position to take charge. On leaving the military service in 1946 I did not return to Boston, but went to the Mount Sinai Hospital in New York City. Doctor Bibring was appointed head of the department and has done a magnificent job.

The problems inherent in the teaching of dynamic psychiatry, although still current, are not new. I had the pleasure during the nineteen thirties of working with Doctors Felix Deutsch and Hermann Blumgart on a project involving the teaching of medical students, interns and residents, subsidized by a grant from the Josiah Macy Jr. Foundation. This paper (Deutsch *et al.*, 1940) was published nearly 25 years ago under the title of "Present Methods of Teaching." I should like to recommend to this audience that they read this paper, if they have not already done so, since many aspects of the discussion today were presented at that time, and some of the recommendations made then are just as relevant today. The teaching of dynamic psychiatry—by which most of us mean the inclusion in our conceptual frame of psychoanalytic concepts—presents many difficulties. Dr. Michaels referred to the fact that he preferred to call himself a psychoanalyst rather than a psychiatrist. On the contrary, I prefer to think of myself as a physician who is a psychiatrist with psychoanalytic training. Since psychiatry is a part of medicine, and dynamic psychiatry has a great contribution to make to all aspects of medicine, we must see to it that the teaching of dynamic psychiatry is not restricted to the residents in psychiatry, but that it becomes a part of the education of medical students and interns and residents who are not going to be psychiatrists. In some ways this may be even more important than the teaching of the potential psychiatrist.

There is a great ferment in the medical educational world today. Conferences are being held, multidisciplinary studies are being made of the medical students and the young graduates, all of which adds up to a great dissatisfaction with the end result. Perhaps the emphasis on basic sciences, leaving out the behavioral sciences, together with the emphasis on techniques and instruments, result in the training of technicians rather than physicians. The psychiatrist, who is a dynamic psychiatrist, is a physician who operationally utilizes not only the basic biological sciences, but also integrates the contribution of the behavioral sciences into the art and science of medicine. It is that teaching contribution which may make the difference between a craft and a profession. One other point—undoubtedly we realize that the dynamic psychiatrist is working in areas which are far from neutral. Because the concepts, themes, and data are highly charged, as Freud has pointed out, they evoke emotional reactions from both the teacher and the student. It is therefore unreasonable to presume that dynamic psychiatry can be presented and accepted as bits of information which are fed in, retained, and retrieved; hence the current emphasis on instrumentation and educational aids as techniques for learning may really be beside the point.

The papers presented today are excellent as practical papers. They have been primarily concerned with tactics employed to bring about this, that, or the other thing. I would be unhappy if each of us left this conference and conducted our teaching in an identical manner. Education, particularly in this area, is not an automatic function. It depends on the teacher, the milieu, the atmosphere, the morale and the student. Each of us, as psychiatrists and psychoanalysts in different situations, may utilize a different timing, training, and content. A certain flexibility is essential. In order to teach, however, one has to know. In order to know, the teacher has to have a firm basic training and experience in the field, and although this alone does not make a teacher, its absence definitely does not permit good teaching.

DR. MICHAELS: Dr. Kaufman emphasizes a point similar to that of Dr. Ewalt's: we are always asking the same questions. However, I would disagree heartily with the statement pertaining to the professional identity of Dr. Kaufman's assertion that first and foremost he is a psychiatrist who secondarily applies psychoanalytic psychology in a psychiatric setting. This leads to the fundamental problem of how one determines one's professional identity, and it raises an issue,

[187]

mentioned by Dr. Gitelson, about the identity crises in psychoanalysis itself. Is psychoanalysis a science in and of itself, or is it a part of psychiatry? On this point, we basically differ. The problem of professional identity is one of the most important questions for all professions.

DR. LINDEMANN: At the close of this thoughtful and comprehensive discussion it remains for me to add one more dimension to the scope of the teaching program so well elucidated by the speakers. The introduction of social science into the field of psychotherapy has brought along the necessity for carefully considering the structure and function of the social systems in which patients are enmeshed. Erikson's work on developmental crises centering on individual life experience has been paralleled by observations of situational crises (Lindemann and Dawes, 1952). These crises constitute precipitous changes in social systems for which the individual was frequently not properly prepared. The changes are then followed by maladaptive responses such as abnormal mourning reactions or puerperal disorders. While the former constitute reactions to the cessation of interaction with a significant other member of the social orbit, the latter represent adjustment to the arrival of a new member of the social orbit, the child just born. Such crises of arrival and departure often form significant opportunities for helpful and preventive intervention, provided that physicians and other caregiving professionals are adequately trained in intervention and in the nature of the psychodynamic reactions during such crises. The professional must know how to evaluate the seriousness of a temporary disorganization and be able to support the patient in marshaling well-adaptive responses to the stress, as well as

[188]

in establishing suitable reorganization of his ego functions, including the search for and the implementation of new roles appropriate to the changed constellation of other persons in the social field.

Not only medical practitioners but also clergymen, teachers, and persons concerned with problems of delinquency and deviance have numerous opportunities to intervene with helpful psychodynamic counseling at the times of critical life experience which are connected with the transition points from one social orbit to another. If well-adaptive responses are solicited and supported, the individual will be in a better position to increase his ego resources. If maladaptive responses and regressive solutions are allowed to crystallize, then the crisis may become a starting point of a self-defeating course of psychological events which often arrive much too late at the door of the psychiatrist.

It is within this context that psychodynamic concepts, and the method of teaching which utilizes material concerned with developmental and situational crises in community life, may make a major contribution in the future to the development of a field of preventive psychiatry.

DR. MICHAELS: When Dr. Lindemann defined himself as a mental-health worker who uses psychoanalytic concepts, I was reminded of something Freud said in 1918: "In psychoanalytic therapy, it is very probable that the large-scale applications of therapy will compel us to alloy the pure gold of analysis freely with the copper of direct suggestion." Whatever form of psychotherapy individuals may select to use, that therapy will be the most effective which is based on the principles of psychoanalysis. Therefore, it is important that the science of psychoanalysis be fostered and strengthened to provide a basic psychology of human behavior which can be applied in all the related disciplines.

* * *

DR. SPIEGEL: I should like to focus on one aspect of Dr. Lindemann's remarks about changing cultural values and practices. This is an extremely important topic, to which we could well devote many hours of discussion.

When a colleague of Dr. Wermer's and Dr. Stock's says, "I am just a pediatrician," he is behaving much like the woman who says, "I am just a housewife." In the woman's case, the tone of apology and self-deprecation is a response to her awareness of her inferiority in respect to the dominant, American, middle-class values. Insofar as these values stress long-range future planning, individual responsibility, and technical mastery in occupational achievements, the housewife can claim only a modest share of esteem in her own eyes and in the eyes of others. When faced with his psychoanalytic colleagues, the pediatrician is apt to believe that he, too, will never be able to attain the skills, the technical mastery, the capacity for taking individual responsibility in the management of psychological problems that the psychoanalyst expects of him—the very skills which the analyst displays with such virtuosity. Like the housewife, he is apt to rank himself as quite low on the scale of values governing success in our society, at least in the area of overlap which he shares with the psychoanalyst.

It seems that it is this type of sensitivity to failure which the work of Drs. Wermer, Stock, and Solnit attempts to correct. Unlike some of the discussants, I do not regard the collaborative approach, which they have so ably demonstrated to us, as a mere tactical maneuver, nor as a drop in the bucket which can never hope to meet the need for imparting psychoanalytic insights to medical colleagues. For the weakness in the dominant, middle-class value system, which is especially evident in the medical professions, is the insistence upon individual responsibility. It is this which produces the feeling of shame or inferiority if one has to consult with, collaborate with, or depend upon others for help with problems of technical mastery over a long period of time. The dominant values lead to the implicit judgment: "After all this time, why haven't you learned to do this on your own?" Looked at this way, if the pediatrician cannot learn quickly and then carry his newly acquired psychoanalytic insights into his everyday practice in an independent fashion, he undergoes a deflation of professional status.

Given the unconscious resistances to psychoanalytic insight, plus the daily pressures of ordinary practice, the expectation of independent performance is unrealistic. Yet, in only a few instances has our medical culture acknowledged the necessity for long-continued collaboration between professions and disciplines. By legitimizing the mutual dependencies growing out of such long-term collaboration and learning, Drs. Wermer, Stock, and Solnit have provided us with a new model for teaching and learning between psychoanalysts and pediatricians. It seems evident that the change in cultural values and practices implied by this model has significance far beyond the particular illustrations offered to us today.

Dr. Onesti, Jr.: I would like to make a few remarks as one who was a member of the early 1957 group that Dr. Solnit

[191]

spoke about. Perhaps in this way I can share with him and with you my lasting impressions from that experience. I was one of the full-time faculty members attending the conference. As director of the pediatric outpatient department at the Yale New Haven Medical Center, I shared teaching and supervisory activities with the practicing pediatricians who attended the conferences. For the purpose of this Symposium (and particularly in response to the question, "Can psychiatry be taught?"), Dr. Solnit has emphasized what he has taught and how he has taught it. He mentioned four areas of psychoanalytic theory upon which he has concentrated and he discussed some case material. He also described the techniques used in moderating group discussions and case presentations. I would like to add to his remarks my own impression as to what it was that made this teaching effective.

The teaching was effective even in the earliest group. As an example of what was taught, Dr. Solnit mentioned that the pediatrician learned how to refer the patient to the child psychiatrist when a diagnosis indicated such referral—in this group, about one in every 10 patients. I would like to point out as a measure of the effectiveness of the teaching that the other nine were not referred but were managed appropriately and successfully by the pediatrician. It seemed to me then, as it does to me now, that the most important factor in making this teaching effective was the active participation of the pediatrician, who brought to the group a problem that had involved and puzzled him. He became active, not only as a student, but more importantly, as a physician; moreover, he became effective as a pediatrician.

Dr. Zetzel has spoken about the importance of having the student play an active role in learning; others have spoken about how to give the medical student and intern (and in many ways these men share the problems of the beginning psychiatrist) an active and effective means of dealing with his feelings of impotence ("I am just a pediatrician"). Dr. Solnit and Doctors Wermer and Stock have described only one aspect of their work with pediatricians. I think that all of us could give examples of how these principles are applied individually or in a group, not only with practicing pediatricians, but also with the pediatric house staff, the residents in child psychiatry, the social workers, and medical students. I think this work fulfills some of the conditions found in the effective teaching of psychoanalytic principles, using close case supervision as discussed by Dr. Bibring. Above all, this type of teaching offers the student a convincing demonstration of applied theory, the importance of which Dr. Bond has so strongly emphasized.

DR. WERMER: The *New Yorker* has a "Department of Correction and Amplification." For the moment, I will call myself the Department of Correction and Amplification and try to amplify or correct some comments by the various speakers. I will not discuss Dr. Solnit's paper beyond saying that I am in wholehearted agreement with him. Next, I want to comment on Dr. Michael's remarks in regard to establishing a therapeutic alliance between teacher and student. Dr. Stock and I have used the word "alliance" in our paper, and not the words "therapeutic alliance," because in teaching we have tried to avoid developing a transference relationship. We wanted to establish a professional alliance between pediatricians and psychiatrists. However, in spite of our best intentions, we have frequently seen the phenomenon of transference in our work.

Let me enlarge upon this. There developed evidence of a

positive group transference to the instructors, namely, Dr. Stock and myself. On the other hand, the transference to our professional identity often became rather negative. Let me illustrate this. The pediatricians in our group often asked us to see in consultation some of their child patients and their families. This referral assumed a special form when the pediatricians insisted that no other psychiatrist but Dr. Stock or Dr. Wermer could ever do justice to the complicated nature of the case. When I heard this, I became conscious of the negative attitude toward our profession. In the eyes of many pediatricians, Dr. Stock and I were acceptable—but our colleagues in psychiatry were not.

My next comment is directed to Dr. John Spiegel: in our thinking we did not neglect the different value systems in pediatrics and psychiatry. It was not included in the paper presented, because it will be discussed extensively by Dr. Zinberg.

In regard to Dr. Ewalt's discussion, I was very much impressed with the material he presented. I agree that we need a small textbook. Our work was not a demonstration project and we did not apply for a grant for such a project. We were sufficiently convinced that our concepts were teachable, and so we applied for and obtained a teaching grant from the National Institute of Mental Health. It is my impression that this panel, in fact, this whole conference, is in some sense a combination of a demonstration project and a scientific lecture.

There is an area in which I differ from Dr. Ewalt—it concerns fishing. I am not much of a fisherman; I am inclined to be a bit bored while waiting for a barracuda; and usually it has been a barracuda that took my bait rather than an edible fish. However, I do feel that if we want to teach basic psychiatric concepts, we have to create within ourselves the patience of a fisherman. We have been trained in this patience throughout our psychoanalytic work. In this work we sometimes sit in our chair and wait for weeks before a patient takes the bait of an interpretation, gets hooked by it, and then carries on with his own introspection.

I want to thank Dr. Gardner for his general discussion. I notice that either his attitude has changed, or that Dr. Stock and I now feel very differently from the way we did when I discussed teaching pediatricians at a meeting of the Judge Baker Clinic more than 10 years ago. When we first started out, we must have had some rather strong emotional reactions and were perhaps more critical of the attitudes of our pediatric colleagues than we are now. At that meeting, Dr. Gardner said, "Dr. Wermer, there is no open season on pediatricians."

Dr. Kaufman, I am very familiar with your papers on teaching psychiatry to nonpsychiatrists. I agree that we have to arouse curiosity and interest in those whom we wish to teach. This can be done in many ways: let me give you an example. I used to make rounds with the pediatric staff in the large old-fashioned wards of the Children's Hospital before it was rebuilt. Once we came to a child who was terrified by the approach of a large group of men in white. Although we merely wanted to talk to the little boy, he began to scream. The technique of approaching him must have occurred to me quite without any rational thinking. While the group stood a few feet away from the bed, I approached the child by walking backward, clicking a cigarette lighter in my hands, while continuing to talk with the rest of the adult group. In two or three minutes, I could feel a tug at my cigarette lighter, which I held behind my back, and could hear some inquiries about it coming from a young voice. This established a friendship between the child and myself, and it certainly aroused his curiosity, because the approach was rather unorthodox. It also created an opportunity to discuss with the pediatricians something about the universal apprehension children feel when they are alone, sick, and suddenly confronted by unknown adults whom they do not regard as friends.

There have been many gratifications and pleasures in our association with this group of pediatricians. Compliments about our skill were always pleasant, but in spite of these, we never forgot that resistances persist. This is something we learn and relearn every day in our practice of psychiatry and psychoanalysis.

Dr. Stock and I discussed one particular patient with the group in great detail. We all agreed that the psychiatric treatment of this child was of tremendous importance. I had kept detailed notes of each session with this girl, and every one in the group seemed convinced that this was primarily a psychogenic problem, and that I was probably saving the girl's life. It was a case of anorexia nervosa. She appeared to be on the verge of irreversible cachexia when she was admitted to a psychiatric hospital and became my patient. This case presentation apparently made quite an impression on our group of pediatricians, for a number of them inquired about the girl months and years after the presentation.

A few weeks ago, near my home, I met one of the pediatricians who had participated in the conference when this case was presented. We greeted each other, regretting that we had not seen each other for some time. Then he asked, "Henry, how is the young girl doing?" I replied, "She is much better. She hasn't gained much more weight, but is

much better, and, you know, it's a long-term proposition."
He then asked, "What are you doing about her mother?" I
answered, "You know, we can't get rid of her. That wouldn't
solve the problem at all. She really isn't that bad anyway."
His next sentence was, "Henry, are you sure that this wasn't
really a case of primary pituitary deficiency?"

Dr. MICHAELS: In the October 1964 issue of the
American Journal of Psychiatry there were three papers devoted to the image of the psychiatrist and one paper on community psychiatry, social psychiatry, and community mental
health work. In one of these papers there is a plea for the
treatment of more patients in the same unit of time than is
now possible, and for the most efficient allocation of our time
and service to a maximum number of people. There is an in-
spirational movement afoot, to reach as many people as possible in the community with the criticism directed to those
psychiatrists who devote their time to relatively few patients
seen only in the office. The development and acceleration of
this community movement can lead to the dilution of clinical
psychiatry, and it threatens the fountainhead from which the
diverse specialized fields of psychiatry draw their vital
resources.

This symposium demonstrates convincingly the significant
effects that a medical psychoanalytic psychology can have on
medical students, psychiatric residents, and physicians in the
community. The more that professional personnel working
in the community are grounded in a scientific psychology,
the better will they carry out their responsibilities. We have
been presented with another image of the psychiatrist, whose
ultimate effect upon the community cannot be gauged by the

amount of time spent and numbers of patients seen, but rather by the pervasive influence that this psychologic point of view can have on patients, medical colleagues, and collaborators in the field of mental health.

PANEL IV: HOUSE OFFICERS

Chairman, ARTHUR F. VALENSTEIN, M.D.

WITHIN THE GENERAL FRAMEWORK of this Symposium, perhaps it will be possible to formulate those aspects which are more specific for the teaching of psychoanalytic medical psychology to house officers, as compared to the teaching of this approach to physicians at other phases in their careers. Of course, the teaching of psychiatric residents is a quite different assignment. I would like to suggest that there is a continuum in the development of the physician and his interest in a medical-psychological point of view. At one end of the scale is the medical student, who, during his first year at least, is perhaps most interested in emotional values and the intricacies of human behavior. His clinical professionalization has barely begun. At the other end of the scale is the physician in the community who has achieved a thorough clinical competency. After he finishes his residency, he begins practice, undertaking full responsibility for his patients, or, and

[199]

this is a somewhat different outcome with somewhat different consequences, he embarks on a teaching-research career in a teaching hospital.

I would like to focus on the process of what I will call, for lack of a better term, the professionalization of the physician. It entails achieving a social role and a self-image of being a well-trained professional person who approaches sick people with an objective scientific perspective, rooted in the study and knowledge of the basic medical sciences. The physician's personal detachment is emphasized in order for him not to be swayed from the soundest medical judgment by sentiments or personal involvements with patients. His scientific detachment and impersonality are a practical necessity, but in excess, they become an occupational hazard in the clinical care of patients. This scientific attitude may reach a peak during the years of internship and residency, when by strongly identifying with highly respected teachers, the house staff may overidealize diagnostic skill and laboratory-oriented methods of patient care. Humanistic influences may not exert their corrective effects until the resident moves into community practice, where he is confronted by the totality of the needs of his patients, and where his patients' dependence can no longer be easily distributed among a corps of physicians and diffused by the institutional framework of the hospital. Only then may his considerations of comprehensive care become more explicit, sometimes giving him a sense of inadequacy, as suggested by Dr. Solnit, when he mentioned that the physicians experienced a throwback to principles of humanistic care which they had forgotten and needed to relearn. I am suggesting that during the training years there may be a definite gradient, a relative diminution of the motivation to learn principles of psychoanalytic medical psychology; for motivation is determined by the inner ideal and the self-expectations of the physician, as well as by external clinical practicalities and exigencies.

We are fortunate in being presented with two articles that complement each other. The first, by Dr. Norman Zinberg, introduces and elaborates on certain principles which might serve as conceptual coordinates for a course on dynamic psychiatry. The second, by Dr. Milton Rosenbaum, is a study of pedagogy at a more empirical level. It will be interesting to see whether one can discern in its rich clinical exemplifications the theoretical values of which Dr. Zinberg speaks.

The Problem of Values in Teaching
Psychoanalytic Psychiatry

NORMAN E. ZINBERG, M.D.

T WO INTERRELATED ISSUES deserve appraisal when considering "The Teaching of Dynamic Psychiatry." First, what
makes up the value system of psychoanalytic psychiatry; and
second, how this value system conflicts with the value systems
of other professional groups and thereby creates problems
for teaching psychoanalytic psychiatry.

In order to discuss these issues, it is first necessary to define
values and the related concepts of morals and ethics—a sur-
prisingly difficult task insofar as values[1] cannot really be defined any more than can truth. Among many other definitions,
Webster defines a value as something (a principle, quality,
or entity) intrinsically valuable or desirable. In a sense, then,
the content of a value depends on the user and the relationship between the user and something outside him

[1] I am indebted to Dr. Peggy Golde for an invaluable discussion differentiating
between the possible statements with which a value statement could be confused.

(Kluckhohn, 1951). To avoid confusion, let me try to spell out what a value is not. "The world is round" is an existential statement which can be a belief, if the person stating it holds it as a cardinal point of religious faith beyond doubt. The same statement can be presented as a hypothesis to be tested; then it yields to the projected measurements which show the world to be slightly elliptical. However, if the person then states that it is better not to be so exact and still likes to say that the world is round, he is making a value statement.

Edward Bibring's (1952) example of the influence of value on perceptions illustrates best how I mean to use the concept.[2] If a soldier, a carpenter, a dendrologist, and an artist look at a tree, they all see the same thing, but conceive of it differently, depending on their value systems. The extent to which they conceive of it as a cover from ambush, material for cabinetry, or as a part of a biological or aesthetic system varies, but when faced with another's view of a tree, they can grasp that different view, as a believer cannot. Nevertheless, the artist's automatic value and concern about the tree as an aesthetic experience influences deeply how he perceives the tree, what he notices about it, the way he thinks and feels when confronted by it, and his description of it to others. In my definition of value, a person's value system is an intrinsic part of his identity as an adult, and whatever the earlier or basic connections to primitive desires may be, it assumes that the complex of motives now operative in the

[2] I was tempted by the word "ideology" to express my meaning as the term is used by Parsons (1951, pp. 353-354), and to a certain extent by Erikson (1958, p. 22), but the confusion about the term and the political and religious implications as described by Bell (1960, p. 370) influenced my decision to stick to the concept "value."

use of his values is largely semiautonomous from their instinctual precursors. To give a contrasting illustration, if someone were to say, "It is good to persecute minority groups," it would be conceived of as a symptom still directly connected to primitive, unconscious motives, and not as relatively autonomous.

When a value carries the connotation of absolute right or wrong, it becomes a moral. According to this definition, a value retains an element of relativity, while a moral does not. Ethics is defined as the translation of a value system into standards or a code of behavior.

Psychoanalysis undoubtedly implies a strong system of values, but little attention has been paid to an explicit codification of them. Heinz Hartmann (1960) in his study of the moral values of psychoanalysis points out that one possible reason for this lack of interest stems from Freud's indifference and essentially pragmatic approach to "ethics" and underlying belief systems unless they related to the psychological study of behavior, although he believed profoundly in ethical behavior.

It is possible that psychoanalytic values remain stronger and more pervasive by not being explicit. It is not my aim to offer a comprehensive study of the values underlying psychoanalytic thought, but rather to identify and describe three values which seem to present problems when teaching members of other medical specialties: (1) psychoanalytic psychiatrists believe that an extensive understanding of a patient's psychological state and its relationship to *all* his life experiences is valuable; (2) in our professional capacity we should not judge or direct our patients morally; and (3) we assume that unconscious feelings which contradict a patient's conscious feelings exist simultaneously with them and should be taken into account. The medical doctor, on the other hand, believes that (1) understanding of a patient's psychological state is important insofar as it relates to the patient's presenting or underlying complaint but is otherwise secondary; (2) physicians should judge and direct their patients in many situations; and (3) the physician usually need not interest himself in anything but the patient's consciously stated feelings.

These two sets of values go beyond the idiosyncrasies of individual physicians and into the basic systems of thought which underlie their identities as psychoanalytic psychiatrists or physicians of other, more physiologically oriented specialties. They go beyond the everyday decisions about what makes for good treatment. No conflict need exist between clinical judgment in an individual case—which may frequently require a therapeutic intervention contrary to certain values—and the retention of a value system. The purpose of this paper is not to criticize the values of psychoanalysts or of other medical specialists, but to ask how these values work in our teaching. If I appear to draw too sharp a distinction between psychological and physical doctors, it must be remembered that such a split is the inevitable result of isolating particular aspects from their natural state where they are surrounded by other elements.

It should be remembered that, in the examples presented, any physician of either group may say correctly that in that instance he would have acted differently. The decision about a specific patient is not important. What is important is to determine how the individual character structures which may have helped determine the choice of profession, the different trainings, and the different needs of our professional functions result not only in our using different theoretical con-

[206]

structs in our work but also different values. For instance, the psychoanalyst, except for the occasion of a suicidal patient, rarely needs to cope with the imminence of death as part of his daily work. In fact many analysts, in discussing their medical school experience of anatomy classes or autopsies, remark how difficult it would be for them to repeat the experience now; now they would be more aware of the depth and intensity of less conscious feelings (requiring quite different defenses) which, as students or house officers, they were able to handle successfully as a joke, by isolation, or by complete lack of awareness. The physicians of many specialties must retain the defenses that enable them to cope with such feelings, and to do so must adopt a system of values which may be incompatible with an insistence upon their knowing as much as possible about all human experiences. This is the sort of thing that goes beyond individual differences, no matter how marked, and into what it means to be a doctor of a particular specialty and how one thinks and feels about what one does.

Before discussing these values, a brief survey of the history of some efforts to teach psychoanalytic principles to physicians might help to establish relevance. Freud and his early followers met with considerable resistance from the medical profession to the great discoveries of psychoanalysis. At the time, a popular psychoanalytic explanation for at least some of the negative reactions to their teaching concerned the nature of the material. Certain ideas such as childhood sexuality, psychoanalysts said, stirred up unconscious defenses which manifested themselves as a conscious feeling of revulsion. This feeling of disgust about certain ideas led to their rejection, and thereby barred from the listener's consciousness any vestiges of his own early, ungratified, and un-

[207]

resolved fantasies. This unconscious response perniciously invaded intellectual judgment, so that psychoanalytic findings in many cases were not received in terms of their logic and clinical verifiability, but were heard through ears conditioned by the defenses of distortion and rejection. As we know, this response to Freud's work caused considerable pain to him and to others. Their understandable solution was to argue that truly to grasp the nature and complexity of the secrets hidden in the depths of the human mind, most people must themselves undergo psychoanalysis. No precise specification was made, however, about which aspects of psychoanalytic thought could, and which could not, be understood without the person's being analyzed.

This pronouncement by leading analysts caused much ill feeling among doctors and those in related professions. Not only was it considered precious and anti-intellectual, but it was also regarded as a kind of circular reasoning. In existing educational institutions, other disciplines, and especially other branches of medicine, spoke of psychoanalysis as dwelling in an ivory tower, asking for special consideration and different rules of procedure for inclusion in the curriculum. Unfortunately for their acceptance in the medical schools, analysts too saw themselves as different. That they should not touch a patient or—until recently—give a prescription, was all too close to an ironclad rule. (Now, perhaps some go too far in the other direction, but that is another problem.)

Gradually things began to change, at least in the United States. American physicians trained in psychoanalysis in Vienna came back eager to tell their colleagues of the wonders they had learned, and particularly World War II gave dynamic psychiatry a chance to show what it had to offer (Zinberg, 1964a). After the war, psychoanalytic institutes

[208]

experienced a great demand to train people who wished to remain within the framework of academic medicine. Under the circumstances, many analysts felt obliged to attempt communication of their principles and underlying theoretical tenets without insisting that such learning be, or be a part of, a therapeutic experience for their nonpsychiatric colleagues. At the same time, physicians of other specialties who had been impressed by dynamic psychiatry, particularly in the armed services, were much more willing to try to listen without prejudice. (I am leaving for another time the discussion of the influence that our mass culture's silly infatuation with psychoanalysis had on this whole process [Zinberg, 1965]). Now began the era of good feeling. Psychoanalysts were appointed to medical school faculties in great numbers; teaching opportunities were opened to them which they accepted. On both sides the attitude which permeated the interspecialty relationships was that men of good will could understand each other's hypotheses if jargon were eschewed on one side and prejudice on the other. An objective evaluation of clinical evidence presented as "scientifically" as possible was to be the prime consideration.

It is my impression that this era now requires reassessment. Unquestionably there have been many gains, but there remain uncertainty about motives, failures in communication and, regretfully, genuine mistrust. The problem before us is the difference between the values of psychoanalysis and those of the other medical specialties, and how that difference represents a barrier, perhaps an insurmountable one, to the teaching of psychoanalytic principles.

Although my impression persists that this conflict of values arises in any relationship between psychological and physical doctors, my primary emphasis will be placed on the problem

[209]

as it relates to the teaching of house officers in a general hospital (Zinberg, 1964b). Their particular stage of development makes them especially suitable subjects for this survey. As medical students, not only the number of facts they must learn, but also the responsibility they have accepted for the life or death of a patient through their supposed knowledge, give rise to fears that often result in psychological rigidity and a narrowing of interests. Their conscience dictates that they must have by their bedsides the *New England Journal of Medicine,* even if unread, rather than *Esquire* (at least they have to be able to say the *New England Journal* is there). The change illustrated by the second-year student's description of a patient as "an old man who talked so much" versus the fourth-year student's "coronary in the second bed from the left" need not be, and in fact usually is not, total: it probably represents an attempt of the student to identify completely with a stereotype of the professional physician. But insofar as this identification interferes with the student's freedom of expression of his own style and an awareness of his own feelings, it acts as a block in learning psychological principles.

When the student gets his degree and becomes a house officer, he is for the first few months of internship, even more anxious and uncertain. Then, more or less suddenly, he finds that he can do his job and has greater control and knowledge than he had suspected. This engenders a degree of relaxation, at which time he shifts from accepting *in toto* what he has been told, to absorbing a basic way of thinking, a system of beliefs that will, in the future, underlie and color all else that he learns. During this period of flux the process of the development of values shows itself clearly.

He is, of course, doing a great many other things during this same period, besides developing a value system, that lead to his final conceptualization of the role of medical doctor and how he sees himself in that role. He learns, for instance, without quite knowing it, a concept of time in relation to illness that differs from specialty to specialty but, once assimilated, is hard to change. Contrast the surgeon's attitude toward this basic dimension with that of the psychoanalytic psychiatrist, and a fundamental difference in outlook becomes apparent. These basic principles are being learned when the house officer has pretty well decided what his future specialty will be. It is a more specific process than that which occurs during medical school, no matter how sure he was at that time about his future choice, because now, with his growing sureness about his competence as a doctor, he really sees himself as ready to learn a specialty and accept the responsibilities that go with it. Therefore, he is making an almost irrevocable choice and committing himself not just to a learned body of material but, in a sense, to a way of life. During this time, house officers become very much concerned about those aspects of their functioning that turn on the values or ethics of their chosen specialty. The intern who will go into psychiatry begins to spend more time with his patients, and in his medical histories emphasizes the past and social history; the future specialist in internal medicine worries about the use of placebos and whether he should treat his own family. These concerns with the less tangible aspects of his identity shape his way of thinking, his values, for the rest of his professional life.

The psychoanalyst's belief that an extensive understanding of a patient's psychological state and its relationship to *all* his life experience is essential, could be said to be the basis of psychoanalysis itself as a therapeutic technique. This value encompasses a wide range of belief in the benefits of under-

NORMAN E. ZINBERG

standing, originating with the analyst himself. The more the
analyst knows about himself, the better prepared he is to treat
patients; the more he knows and understands about the patient, the better it is for the patient in any circumstance;
finally (within the limitations of clinical judgment, correct
timing, and Anna Freud's (1946) delineation of repression as
a necessary concomitant of successful development), the more
the patient understands about himself, the better his chances
for recovery. In a discussion of the interaction of psychoanalytic and general medical values, it is the understanding of
the patient by the doctor that concerns us.

We explain this to other doctors, in part, by pointing out
that it is relatively easy to see in one patient certain corre-
spondences with others. And, although we know that at different times in his life different conflicts are uppermost, we can
usually get a pretty fair idea, in an interview or two, of what
conflict is uppermost at that particular time. However, a genuine understanding of how the derivation and use of this person's conflict differs from those of other people, how he is
unique and special, requires a careful, searching consideration of as many of his thoughts and feelings as is possible,
which we must fit together into a coherent whole that will
stand for this one person.

This is the doctrine of inclusion (Zinberg, 1963). The other specialties of medicine, despite protestations to the contrary, work primarily by the process of exclusion. A series of
possibilities, usually ranging from the more to the less severe,
is considered until either a diagnosis is fixed upon or anything that might be dangerous to the health of the patient has
been reasonably excluded. Bits and pieces of an unusual finding can be overlooked if the important and pathognomonic
findings are negative. Here the psychiatrist and his medical

[212]

colleague see matters differently. In a general hospital, the effect of their differing views presents itself when a psychiatrist is asked for a consultation about a medical patient. The question the psychiatrist is asked about the patient—"Is this particular illness organic or functional?"—may be answered on the basis of a relatively brief study. He may say that the absence of a precipitating factor, the lack of any previous history of this type of psychological response, and the quality of the patient's anxiety about the illness itself, indicate a high probability that the etiology is organic. But he will further inform the referring physician that, if he wishes to manage this patient to his best advantage, he must know more about the extent of his reaction to his symptoms and about the factors that led him to consider in the first place that the illness might be functional.

It is at this point that the psychiatrist and the medical man lose a degree of contact, not because the medical man disagrees, for he doesn't entirely. He thinks, "Yes, we must know more, but we have ruled out something of great importance, and now we must do four tests and five X-rays to rule out these several possible diagnoses, and when we have finished with these, we can come back to the now relatively nonurgent factor of this man's emotional state." For the medical man it is not urgent because it is not directly contributory to the patient's disease. The psychiatrist at this point may say, "Yes, those tests are of the greatest importance, but the way in which the patient is approached about them, the extent to which he understands what is going on, are equally urgent." To establish a good relationship with the patient that will achieve optimal cooperation both verbally and emotionally, the physician must find out a little more about how the patient views what is happening.

[213]

Here is what looks like no more than a difference of opinion about which procedure comes first, with each party recognizing the validity and importance of the other's position. But I submit that there is an essential clash of values reinforced by different methods of training and practice. For the medical man, once it is reasonably established that the illness is primarily organic, the fact that the patient reacted excessively is treated as a factor to be put on his list and dealt with in its time. For the psychiatrist, it is part of the whole fabric of what is going on and has to be included with all else that is done. What at first may appear quantitatively as a difference in emphasis emerges qualitatively as a growing lack of communication between two doctors concerned with the well-being of their patient; the psychiatrist often feels that he has not been able to convey his specific knowledge of what is going on in that patient—and certainly not the general principles that underlie this understanding—so that the medical man can have them to refer to in his future interactions with that patient. This problem of communication then shows itself as a resistance by one or both of the doctors and can take several forms.

The most important point of disagreement—that the medical man is not genuinely convinced that more knowledge of the patient's emotional state is vital unless something specific in the diagnostic study during the hospital course makes it so, while the psychiatrist can hardly think in any other way—rarely comes directly to light. Both leave such a case with a slightly greater question about how much they have to offer each other. The medical man most often decides that time is of the essence, and that to do what the psychiatrist suggests would delay the necessary diagnostic tests or would demand more of his day than he could possibly commit regularly to any one patient. (The use of time as a rationalization has been dealt with convincingly by John F. Reichard, 1964). The analyst all too often decides that perhaps the patient and doctor would both be better off working things out between them, doing what comes naturally without outside interference, and he either slowly or abruptly withdraws from the case.

The second value to consider—the belief that we as analysts cannot and should not judge or, in many instances, direct our patients—contains the essence of the stereotyped view of psychoanalysts. In the deepest sense, judgment occurs in every human interaction, and in this total sense, the analyst does judge his patients. But he does not judge them by conventional moral standards: he "judges" and values the patient's understanding of himself and his taking responsibility for his own choices and decisions. We direct patients too, but so differently from the usual medical doctor that the whole concept is changed. When we say, "Tell us your thoughts and fantasies," we give directions similar to the request for a medical history of symptoms. But after the history is obtained and a diagnosis is made, the medical doctor can prescribe penicillin or some other drug. If the patient refuses to cooperate in watching his regimen, someone else can help.

The analyst cannot prescribe understanding. The patient must accept a different sort of responsibility, which leads to a value that emphasizes his freedom from direction. It should be understood that different analysts' personalities, styles, and philosophies—and even confusion on this subject—vary enough so that their answers to a question about the direction of a patient may differ. However, analysts generally would agree with the central concept that the passing of a moral judgment on a patient's behavior, thoughts, or feelings is not their function. Judging implies that there is a right way

[215]

and a wrong way. But certainly the medical doctor must direct his patients. In many instances of physical disease, there is a standard which can be validated and the job of the medical doctor is to find the right way and indicate it to his patient: for example, to remain healthy a diabetic must take insulin and stay on a diet. The psychoanalyst's patients usually complain of less concrete ailments than diabetes, and the job of the psychoanalyst is to help his patients to permit themselves a genuine choice which is not overdetermined by unconscious elements, while not making the choice for them; e.g., even after a homosexual has come to understand that the feelings that have led to close relationships with all people are unnecessarily terrifying, he may continue to be a homosexual.

Our two brief examples lead us to a maze of great complexity. The stereotype of the psychoanalyst as a person who permits and even condones behavior which is at best immoral and at worst antisocial goes back to Freud's earliest work on the subject of sexuality. The misunderstanding of the psychoanalytic concept of responsibility leads the medical man to see the analyst as overpermissive and unsure about questions of behavior which affect the well-being of the patient and sometimes that of his family and friends. If the diabetic patient does go off his diet, the physician unhesitatingly condemns his behavior as wrong and looks for a way to set it right. In extreme examples the issue is clear-cut; but if, for example, the diabetic is an adolescent who wants to drink beer with the rest of his gang, and the doctor and the analyst must determine at just what point the physical and at just what point the psychological well-being of the patient must be served, disagreements occur. The ostensible difference of opinion about the proper treatment often masks the medical doctor's feeling that the psychoanalyst, when he expends so much thought

[216]

on how the incident fits into the patient's personality structure, his time of life, and certain unresolved emotional conflicts, unnecessarily postpones instructing the patient about his proper conduct and, in a word, indulges him. Here the issue is hazy, and the difference in function between the medical doctor and the analytic psychiatrist—represented by their differences in values—may determine their therapeutic recommendations.

With the homosexual, the problem of judgment is clearer. Often when a family or the patient himself recognizes the existence of this problem, he is first, especially if he is young, taken to a medical doctor. The usual response of the medical doctor (if he doesn't wash his hands of the patient by telling him that he must "cut it out" or that he should just learn to live with the disease) is to investigate and attempt to eliminate any physical reason for the aberration, such as undescended testicles, endocrinological disturbance, etc. If no organicity is found, psychiatric referral often follows. By unquestioningly accepting the homosexual behavior as an aberration to be cured, the medical doctor reflects our society's values, and conveys to the patient a judgment which must have moral connotations.

The analytic psychiatrist, when faced with the same patient, would from the beginning entertain the possibility that for this particular patient an adjustment as a homosexual may be preferable to the other possibilities open to him. Even though the psychiatrist knows that in this culture social pressure would overwhelmingly condition the choice once unconscious pressures were relieved, he recognizes that a choice remains, and avoids judging or directing the patient. In order to ensure that this distinction is more than a purely semantic one, during the course of a treatment he must frequently, without interdiction, accept behavior that would trouble most medical doctors. But it is not in the acceptance that the value difference lies as much as in the initial approach. For the medical doctor it is natural to judge the homosexuality as wrong and to try to eliminate it; in doing so, the physician is following his belief that he must judge and direct his patients. In fact, he often resents here, as much as with the diabetic patient, the psychiatrist's indirect and circuitous approach to the problem and feels that it is an implicit, obscure criticism of himself.

Such criticism is usually not intended. Not only does the psychiatrist recognize that supplying a regimen is second nature to a physician, but also that patients request and often demand advice from their physicians which is tantamount to a moral judgment. The analytic psychiatrist himself receives the same demands from patients, who insist on attempting to mesh the stereotype of psychoanalysis as condoning immorality and weakness as illness with a view of the analyst as a guardian of conventional morality. They insist that his ideas of mental health and illness, of stability and inhibition, of control and impulses, are merely new words fitted to old ideas and that he has become the judge in a new guise. Consequently, it is not the analyst's disapproval of the medical doctor's "judgments" which disrupts communication as much as their different ways of perceiving problems.

Another way of illustrating these different views involves the question of conveying to the patient that he has done something well. Both the medical man and the psychiatrist are usually chary about praising the patients directly, but for different reasons. Although the analyst avoids moral judgments, he certainly has many, often ill-defined, ideas of competence even in psychiatric treatment. Both he and the patient may know that in a particular session certain conflicts are especially clearly delineated—that is, it is a "good" session. But if the psychiatrist were consistently to tell the patient that particular sessions are good sessions and he has done something right, then by direct implication other sessions are bad and he has done something wrong. The psychiatrist would become a judge, and the patient would search for other moral judgments. For this reason analysts try as neutrally as possible merely to point out to the patient that one choice has been made over another. As a result the patient is made aware that another choice was realistically possible, even if he could not consider it at that time. We do not say that his choice was a bad one or an immoral one or a weak one. We show him, if we can, what motives determined his decision.

The medical doctor prescribes a regimen that he considers good for the patient, and expects the patient to follow it. When the routine is followed, praise is unnecessary because the patient has only done what was agreed upon as proper. If he does not follow the routine, he has done something that is clearly wrong, and both doctor and patient agree that he must answer for it. The medical doctor's concern for the motives behind the patient's behavior is much less than his concern with what the patient does. Very often and understandably, even in matters concerning the patient's emotional life, medical doctors will attempt to work out a problem with a patient and offer advice. If the patient finds himself unable to act on this advice, he will feel that he is wrong and often his doctor will agree. Here again both psychiatrist and medical doctor have performed admirably according to their different value systems, but communication about such differences becomes difficult.

This difficulty in communication, based on the different

[219]

value systems, often shows itself when the medical doctor attempts to apply what he hears from the psychiatrist. The analytic psychiatrist may say that certain unpleasant, but repressed, feelings—anger in the diabetic, perverse sexual impulses in the homosexual—seek some form of discharge, and that if the patients could recognize and talk about those feelings, they might avoid unnecessary self-destructive behavior. The medical man accepts this, returns to the patients in question, and tells them to express their feelings, that in fact it is essential for them to do so. Very often in such instances the psychiatrist finds that in the interchange with the medical doctor the neutrality which he attempted to convey in his statement has been lost and has become a different way of thinking about the same subject. It was not resistance, nor was he actually misunderstood; rather, the subtle transformation of a value into a moral occurred because of a different system of thought and different functions. The medical doctor reports that the diabetic adolescent "clammed up" and was resentful, and that the homosexual went into elaborate details about his sexual activity. In neither case was the next step clear to the doctor, and so both patient and doctor were disappointed. The doctor asks, "What happened? How is what I did wrong?" The psychiatrist tries to explain that such discussions, to be useful, can't be forced but must occur when the patient is "ready," and that the patient who goes to a medical doctor does not expect the "talking treatment" he would expect if he went to a psychiatrist. What the medical doctor did was not wrong; but the psychiatrist, because of different training, a different underlying attitude in approaching the patient, and a different response from the patient, does more than ask the patient to reveal feelings: he also helps the patient put these feelings into a perspective that includes the

[220]

rest of his life. And he offers to show the medical man how he can do the same with great effort and further learning.

All too frequently the discussion stops where it began. The medical doctor, armed with a value system that prepares him to deal with the harsh realities of life and death, finds the vague conception of "ready" unsatisfactory and in a way detrimental to his basic function, which involves judging and directing. The psychoanalytic psychiatrist has an almost infinite tolerance of human differences and must, therefore, as part of his function, reject judging his patient's behavior as right or wrong.

The third value to be discussed clearly overlaps and depends on the other two. The belief that unconscious feelings which contradict a patient's conscious feelings exist simultaneously and should be taken into account is important only in a system of thought which is based on inclusion; and attitudes toward judging and directing a patient will differ according to the estimate of what active feelings and ideas in a person need to be considered. The acceptance by psychoanalysts of this value seems total, because underlying it are two basic psychoanalytic theoretical constructs: ambivalence —the simultaneous existence of different, and even opposite, feelings about anything worth caring about—and a dynamic unconscious. For analysts, the capacity to doubt and still act with resolution and spontaneity—that is, to tolerate ambivalence—is a miracle to be exercised all the days of our lives. We find no parent so loving of a child that there is not, at the same time, a particle of hate or envy of that same child. However, we do not regard that particle of hate as the fatal flaw in a perfect love; rather, we respect the strength and even the nobility that goes into the capacity to tolerate the hate and act on the love and goodwill. In believing in absolute love no

[221]

more than we do in absolute faith, we stand against conventional morality and the entire romantic tradition of the Western world. More than that, we stand against the yearning of every person to experience a total feeling which contains no hint of nagging uncertainty.

The psychoanalyst's unceasing awareness of ambivalence is related to the acceptance of a dynamic unconscious, one of the five theoretical constructs on which psychoanalysis could truly be said to stand or fall (Rapaport and Gill, 1959). Psychoanalysts postulate a part of the mind where contradictory ideas exist simultaneously, although the ideas and the unacceptable feelings associated with some of them are refused consciousness, sometimes transiently, sometimes permanently. The psychoanalyst does not maintain that these different and opposite feelings about the same thing are continuously available to anyone, but that these feelings continue their activity and their effect on the person whether conscious or not.

This value of the concept of an unconscious becomes so complete, so much second nature in psychoanalytic psychiatrists, that they are often unaware that their medical colleagues do not entirely share it. Very often, when sitting in on conferences involving medical doctors and psychiatrists, I am reminded of an interchange between two very famous analysts during a clinical case presentation. The presentor on two or three occasions used the word "obviously." The other analyst finally said, "X, when you say 'obviously,' I think you mean that anyone who doesn't agree with you is a fool." That incident occurs to me frequently in joint conferences between analytic psychiatrists and physicians of other specialties, when I hear analysts starting to explain the conflict behind the patient's nonobservance of a medical regimen, or commenting on less obvious, at least relatively less conscious, ideas or feelings that they contend are active. This perennial decision to question the patient's statements, and to deduce many things that are unsaid, often strikes the physician as confusing and unnecessary. In fact, it is as if the medical man hears the psychiatrist constantly saying that the patient doesn't feel what he says he feels, but only "really" feels what he is unaware of or denies.

The problem is illustrated by the situation in which the psychoanalyst tells the patient and the doctor that the patient has feelings of which he is unaware. An excellent example for our discussion would be the patient who presents himself at the hospital before surgery and, when asked how he is, replies that he feels fine. If asked whether he is worried about the operation, he answers that he likes and trusts his doctor and prefers to let the doctor do the worrying. The psychiatrist, when confronted by this patient, says that the patient conceals great anxiety, and that his well-being would be best served if he could face some of his psychic discomfort before the procedure takes place. This sort of insistence on our knowledge of the inner life of a person goes beyond that which tests and X-rays and operations can tell us, beyond and even directly against what the person himself knows and says, and represents a position entirely different from that of the physician. The medical doctor takes a history and decides whether it is reliable. If it is not reliable, he goes elsewhere for his information; if it is reliable, he accepts it. To him it seems as if the psychiatrist never accepts what a patient says, never trusts the patient, and it is almost as if the psychiatrist himself, in his search for dark and complex motives and conflicts, becomes suspect.

The psychoanalyst regards his search for more understanding of the patient's reactions not as suspicious but as natural, and, in the long run, therapeutic and perfectly consonant with his thinking about the nature of man. Complex, opposite feelings seem usual to him. But the medical doctor is more likely to feel that the psychoanalyst mistrusts the patient.

This particular problem results in even greater confusion when the psychiatrist says, as he often does, that one purpose of understanding the patient in depth is to promote greater trust between the doctor and his patient. The medical doctor, assuming that there is no reason to interest himself in other than the patient's consciously stated feelings, finds ridiculous, without a specific indication, the psychiatrist's position that the doctor must question the patient's stated trust in him in order for the patient to trust him.

The problem lies not only in such obvious semantic abuses and other flaws in communication; the psychiatrist's insistence on an awareness of feelings unknown to the patient, and often in such contrast to those known, seems almost to be a claim of prescience, and the medical doctor feels that this claim of deeper knowledge carries with it a claim of superiority which he cannot help resenting.

My impression, strengthened each year by work with physicians, continues to be that the psychoanalytic psychiatrist has not fully understood how thoroughly his thinking—shaped by his personality, his experiences with psychiatric patients, and his rigorous training, which accentuates an interest in motivation, differences, conflicts, and dynamics—differs from that of his medical colleagues. What is more, when I try to consider carefully the value system implicit in psychoanalytic theory, or at least in the attitudes of psychoanalysts as they approach their patients, I become aware of the considerable evidence that the more explicit of their values are indeed ambiguous and troublesome to psychoanalytic doctors themselves. A consideration of what psychoanalysts "truly" believe of their ambivalence, would not be fair or helpful at this point and would only confuse my present aim, which is to clarify somewhat the difficulties in understanding and communication which can arise between psychoanalytic psychiatrists and other doctors.

Where does such clarification take us? Insofar as it suggests certain limits to teaching programs aimed at physicians whose value systems are fixed, insofar as it suggests where medical students and especially house officers should question their attitudes about being doctors, it has implications for medical education. Many people feel that the recent generations of medical graduates, more thoroughly exposed to psychoanalytic thinking, have narrowed the gap between the thinking of the medical doctor and the analytic psychiatrist. However, I still pose as a problem and as a fact that, until the value systems of these two groups—the medical doctors and the psychological doctors—are charted, important limits to communication will be imposed, not by unconscious resistance, not by lack of intellectual competence or goodwill, but by differing values.

Issues Raised in Teaching Psychological Medicine to Medical Students, Medical Residents, and Family Physicians

MILTON ROSENBAUM, M.D.,
THEODORE JACOBS, M.D.,
and SANFORD OXENHORN, M.D.

FOR THE PAST FOUR YEARS, members of our department at Albert Einstein have been engaged in teaching principles of psychological medicine to groups at three levels of training: junior medical students, medical and neurological residents, and family physicians. A comparison of our experiences with these groups soon revealed problems in teaching which, while overlapping in some areas, were nevertheless peculiar to each group, and which related to their different levels of professional maturation.

Our programs for the student and resident groups were somewhat different. In our student teaching, a psychiatrist worked with groups of four students throughout their first clinical year, rotating with them as they moved from service to service. Teaching sessions were held once a week for an hour and a half, during which time the students were encouraged to bring up any patient or problem that interested

[226]

them. Following a brief presentation, the patient was interviewed, first by the instructor, later by the students, and much time was reserved for a discussion of the issues raised in the session—discussions which covered the range of student concerns, from the anxiety felt by students in posing as doctors to the psychological issues raised by the dying patient, and to the care and management by attending physicians.

The resident groups also met weekly for an hour and a half throughout the year, and here too the structure of the sessions was open-ended, so that the residents could bring up any problem that interested them. There was, however, no rotation into specialty areas. Both teaching sessions were supervised by the senior author in a joint weekly meeting of the instructors.

The teaching sessions for family physicians were conducted with a group of Health Insurance Plan physicians (full-time internists and pediatricians) attached to Montefiore Hospital, New York City. On the average, about 15 physicians attended the weekly seminars on a voluntary basis. The format of the sessions was as follows: a brief (five minutes) presentation of a patient was followed by a half-hour interview by the instructor (M. Rosenbaum), who was observed by the group through a one-way screen. However, in the past two years all the interviews behind the one-way screen have been carried out by the patient's physician. The interview was then discussed at some length.

In the first year of our program at Albert Einstein there were two groups, a student group composed of four volunteers interested in psychiatry, and a group of three medical residents who had officially volunteered for the program, but whose arms had been gently twisted by the medical department to do so. The differences in these groups were striking.

The student group met in an atmosphere of informality and free exchange of ideas, with genuine enthusiasm for the sessions. Often two or three students competed to present patients, and the discussions ranged far and wide. The resident group remained formal throughout and tended to be strictly businesslike in the sessions which often began late or were canceled by the group because of the pressure of other duties. Work with the residents, in fact, became so discouraging that we were ready to abandon the project as inoperable. The residents seemed so little motivated and their resistances so high, that we wondered whether we were in error in believing that such a program had any value at all for them.

To our surprise, in the second year the picture began to change. This time the student group was selected at random from students beginning their clerkships in psychiatry. Now the resistance in the student group was strong. The students felt discriminated against. They complained that they were being subjected to a program whose worth they seriously doubted, while their fellow students went scot-free. They were suspicious that they were being placed under surveillance by the psychiatry department, and that they were being punished for critical attitudes toward psychiatry in their first two years. The initial meetings were held in an atmosphere of distrust and resentment, which only gradually gave way, as the students developed positive feelings for the instructor and began to identify with him. The changes that took place in the subsequent resident groups will be taken up in later pages.

Issues Raised in Student Teaching

In our experience with medical students over the past several years, we have gained some understanding of the central issues in teaching psychological medicine at this level of training by use of the preceptor method. The student at the beginning of his clinical work is faced with the triple-threat task of maintaining his self-esteem with patients and staff, gaining the approval of his teachers, and containing the anxieties aroused by his first contact with patients. Such experiences as examining the body, witnessing birth, learning intimate details of a patient's life, or performing painful procedures all serve to mobilize latent conflicts that must be mastered. The anxieties raised by the dying patient, the paralyzed or aged patient, as well as the sexually attractive patient, call forth adaptive responses that, while highly individual, have been traditionalized by the time-honored role of the clinical clerk. In asking the student to involve himself with the psychological aspects of medical illness, we may appear to him to challenge the equilibrium he has attained. In medical-student culture, self-esteem often rests on being sharp, on knowing the clinical entities, and on being keen in picking up physical signs.

When we ask a student to obtain psychological information, he often feels thrown into deep water, first, because he is unaware of how to obtain the information, and second, because he has no clear idea of what to do with it. The material we elicit may interest him, but it puzzles and confuses him in a way, whereas learning that a patient has chest pain on exertion does not. He often feels guilty about his voyeuristic impulses, particularly when obtaining a sexual history, and he may compensate by trying to offer the patient some reassurance about his condition—to do some therapy, as it were—but that effort may bring with it the uncomfortable doubt as to whether his words really helped or perhaps may have injured his patient. It is safer for him not to get involved. Unless we give the student adequate preparation for a psychological approach to patients, we are in the position of giving him a stethoscope and asking him to examine a heart without training him to use the instrument. Thus we would put him in the feared position of looking like an amateur in front of his patients, his colleagues, and himself. Ironically, therefore, while we are attempting to increase the student's confidence in his abilities by extending the range of his knowledge, we may, in his eyes, be decreasing it.

By concerning himself with psychological principles, the student may also run the risk of being thought of as different, an outsider in the real world of medicine, and he may be dubbed a "psychiatrist" by teachers or fellow students. Many students, while interested in the emotional life of a patient, will avoid revealing this interest for fear of being type-cast in this way. One of our most difficult students was a young man whose cynicism about the program knew no bounds. Hardly a session went by when he did not open the discussion by asking why psychiatrists were so full of fantasy, what they had against the scientific method, and how he could get out of the program. When it was his turn to present a patient, he discussed the case of a homeless 85-year-old woman who had entered the hospital in heart failure and was to be sent to a nursing home. During the subsequent interview, the patient revealed that the student had been coming to see her every day and that she had spent many hours chatting with him about old times when she was a popular young girl. Just before the group left the room, the patient thanked the student for bringing her a flower that morning.

For many students, however, the method of coping with the anxieties aroused by their patients is to avoid them, a defensive behavior in which the medical faculty is often an ally. In most clerkships, the student is expected to take a routine history, do a physical, perhaps perform some laboratory procedures—and there his responsibility to his patient ends. In most medical-school training the student is not required to talk with his patient. He knows that family and emotional problems rarely turn up on ward rounds and certainly not in examinations. Also, the fact that the patient is hospitalized and that whatever psychological problems may arise during his stay can be handled by a resident, nursing staff, or psychiatric consultant, makes keeping one's distance easier for the junior clerk as compared to the senior student working in the outpatient department where the patient views the student as the doctor, and the emotional problems that arise cannot in good conscience be so easily avoided.

In our student groups, as contrasted with the resident sessions, the instructor became much more the preceptor, to whom the students could express their fears in working with patients. In the permissive and informal atmosphere of the small group, the students could bring up their fear of getting angry at patients, of hurting them, or of being humiliated by them. They talked about patients whom previously they had avoided. Early in our sessions a student presented a 70-year-old man with advanced gastric cancer who had a fistulous opening that was draining foul-smelling material. The students entered this man's room with noticeable hesitation and kept at a distance from his bedside until the instructor shook hands with the patient and started to speak to him. Later it was learned that the house staff rarely entered this patient's isolated room on rounds, and that none of the students had ever been in it. They had clearly used this group session to have the instructor lead them to this dying man with a stinking wound, whom they had fearfully avoided. In our experi-

[231]

ence, the student's freedom to express his anxieties in an un-critical setting is crucial to the learning process. Gradually the instructor's attitude, not only toward sick patients but also toward the students themselves, becomes integrated with the professional self-image. It is this process of identification which, particularly at this stage of training, is so important in developing psychological sensitivity in the student.

ISSUES RAISED IN THE RESIDENT GROUPS

In our first year with the medical residents, the meetings tended to assume a formal atmosphere, much like a group of residents presenting their patient to a psychiatrist for consultation. There was little discussion of the doctor-patient relationship or of the doctor's own feelings. The frequent absences, the canceled sessions, and the group's request for an early termination of the sessions led both the instructor and his supervisor to infer a lack of interest in the program. However, in a discussion held with their own director of resident training, the group members reported that they had found the experience, which was the first for both the medical service and the psychiatric instructor, extremely worthwhile. Two meetings especially impressed them. In the first, the instructor had interviewed a young man with ulcerative colitis, whose clinical course was steadily deteriorating. The members were struck by his ability to obtain fresh, relevant, historical information. Further, when he formulated the areas of conflict in this patient and made specific recommendations for his management, the young man began to improve. The residents now felt there was some practical value to the sessions.

In the other session which they reported to their faculty member, a young man on the neurology service was pre-

[232]

sented because of his bizarre behavior, strange thoughts, and inability to walk. The chief of service had made the diagnosis of a conversion-reaction psychosis. The instructor noted classical signs of an organic mental state, as well as scanning speech and ataxia. He suggested that the patient be studied for multiple sclerosis. This turned out to be the correct diagnosis. The residents were impressed by the medical skill of the instructor, who in turn became aware of how important it was for him, as a security measure, to impress the medical residents with his competence as a physician and teacher.

Two suggestions of the members of the first group were put into effect for all subsequent groups. The meetings convened on the medical wards, rather than in the instructor's office on the psychiatric floor of the hospital; and after the instructor had had an opportunity to demonstrate interviewing technique, the resident members did the interviewing in later sessions.

With the second group of residents, it was apparent that the stiff consultation atmosphere of the first year was no longer present. The residents spoke of their feelings toward patients, of the patients' reactions to them as doctors, and they selected typical medical patients for presentation because they intrigued or puzzled them. It was a consistent observation that their selection of patients revealed their own anxieties. In the third meeting, one of the residents presented a 48-year-old woman, nearly blind and uremic, who was in a state of chronic heart failure with periarteritis nodosa. The resident sensed that she was aware of the downhill course ahead and that she wanted to ask him about her future. He had never given her an opportunity of raising the question. During the interview with the instructor, she described her overwhelming sense of loss, her fear of helplessness and abandonment. She wanted to know from her doctor, "What will become of me?" In the discussion that followed, the instructor was able to point out to the residents that he too felt quite helpless with this patient, but he realized that in part it was because he had identified with her. He explained that while the doctor always hopes he can offer a cure, he can help a dying patient as well. In this case the patient needed to know that her doctor understood her suffering and would respond to her pleas for help. The physician could also be helpful by correcting certain distorted fantasies she had about her illness. The instructor also noted how often the doctor's conception of a patient's fears is not at all what the patient truly fears.

An important session for this group centered on the change of ward assignments. At the time of the switch in house staff, the members of the group elected to make rounds in order to learn what effect their departure had on their patients. In the discussion they also brought out their own feelings about leaving the patients with whom they had been working. We felt that this experience was instrumental in permitting the residents in future sessions to express more openly their personal reactions to patients.

The members of the third group took somewhat longer than their predecessors to feel comfortable about discussing their own feelings, but they largely followed the pattern of the second year. A special characteristic of this group was its ability to deal openly with sexual problems in patients.

We considered the reasons for the disparity between the observations made in Group I and all subsequent resident groups, including that in neurology. We recognized first that the teacher's role was crucial in shaping the course of each year's program. The teaching of Group I was the first such

[234]

experience for the instructor (S. Oxenhorn). Further, it was his first opportunity to return to a medical setting following his departure from medicine to train in psychiatry. His uncertainty regarding his own position between these two disciplines, his unsure feeling about the value of such a teaching exercise, and other conflicts within himself were dealt with by establishing a rather formal, structured atmosphere. With further experience, he was able to create a more relaxed environment, in which a free exchange of ideas could take place.

A second important factor was the attitude of the medical staff. In the first resident group, the members in time disclosed that they were swimming against the current of popular opinion. The other residents who were not members repeatedly questioned their presence in the group and teased them about it. Furthermore, the faculty member who had advocated their joining the group was not the most popular figure.

Once Group I was completed, all three of its members became more important people on the house staff. One member immediately became chief resident, and the other two were destined to do likewise the following year. These latter two became strong advocates of the group and often spoke about it to their colleagues. The climate on the medical service changed. By the time Group III was being formed, eight of a possible 12 residents volunteered to join the group. It was clear that what a respected chief resident thought to be worthwhile was now sought after, rather than ridiculed.

Differences between Medical and Neurological Resident Groups

The differences between the medical and neurological resident groups were also interesting. The first group on the neurology service was composed of the chief resident, one second-year resident, and three first-year residents. This was a departure from the more uniform medical resident groups, and it is not clear just what effect such a mixture of hierarchical levels had on the cohesiveness of the members. The chief resident admitted that he felt on the spot, and that he had to put in a good showing for the others. At first we thought his presence would so inhibit the group, and would result in so much self-consciousness, that we suggested he drop out. However, the other residents became very resentful of his exclusion, and because of their feeling he was reinstated.

This was again the first time the instructor had worked with a neurology group, and subsequent experience may modify our view of teaching in this setting. However, the differences we found between the medical and the neurological resident groups impress us as having been instructive.

The personalities and interests of the neurology residents were quite unlike those of their medical colleagues. They were very much interested in the brain as a machine, and were less closely involved with their patients. Their use of intellectualization as a defense was striking. For the neurology residents, the concept of the role of the doctor was that of a recorder of data rather than that of a healer. For example, on the mental-status examination they were surprised when the instructor attempted to orient a disoriented patient, or to reduce his anxiety and then retest a given function in which the patient had fared poorly.

These attitudes on the part of the residents seemed to us in part reflections of the necessary defenses that the neurologist requires to cope with his clinical work. Since so many of his patients are unresponsive, either brain-damaged or stuporous, and he can neither effect a change nor interact with them as human beings, his major gratification must come from his developing skill as a diagnostician. The medical residents, by contrast, have a different group of patients to work with; while they have had their share of intractable cases, they also commonly enjoy the rewards of a therapeutic success. It may be, too, that modern neurology, because of its strong emphasis on the conceptual and theoretical issues of mind and brain, attracts men to whom intellectual satisfaction is most important.

Unlike their medical colleagues, the neurologists did not unite on issues of common feelings, but rather on the fact that they were all in neurology and therefore had a common interest in certain specific topics. They initiated many seminar-like discussions of basic philosophic issues, which included such questions as: What is this thing called mind? What part of any given patient's pathologic picture is physical and what part is functional? They also requested seminars on specific topics, with the group reading the appropriate literature. These were among the topics included: denial of illness, the euphoria of multiple sclerosis, the thought disorder in schizophrenia, depression, and the psychoanalytic concept of the mental apparatus. The neurologists began the sessions with the view that the physical and the psychological were sharply compartmentalized. It took repeated discussions and a prolonged process of gradual change, with occasional crises of uncertainty, before any member could employ the concept of a dynamic interaction between mind and body.

The Role of the Supervisor

The supervisor of the program (M. R.) met weekly with the course instructors. In these sessions each instructor had an opportunity to give an account of his previous session with the medical students or residents. Occasionally the supervisor discussed some particular clinical aspect of a case, but for the most part he focused on the difficulties of the instructor in the teaching exercise and repeatedly emphasized the following points:

1. The anxieties, blocks, and resistances of the teachers appeared to be as important to the learning process as those of the students. As an example, one instructor, well-trained in medicine as well as in psychiatry, repeatedly reported that his group of students alternately presented him with either classical medical problems or a primarily psychiatric patient. It soon became clear that the instructor had a conflict about his own identity as a psychiatrist and had not yet given up his desire to be known as a qualified internist. Thus his particular anxiety in this teaching exercise was allayed by his unconsciously signaling to the students that he enjoyed discussing complicated medical problems.

2. The identification of the teachers with the students was also emphasized. Time and again the instructors reported incidents in which the students were highly critical of the behavior and attitudes of the house and attending staffs. Although some of these derogatory accounts might have had some basis in truth, it became apparent that the psychiatric instructors enjoyed hearing such reports and tended to side with the students in their disparagement of medical colleagues. The supervisor had to point out that what appears to the student as lighthearted behavior, on the part of the house staff, in the face of the dying patient, or as cold, inconsiderate, and sadistic attitudes in the surgical wards and the operating rooms, or as cruel and disrespectful handling of the helpless comatose patient, may unfortunately

[238]

be true. More often than not, however, the observed physician really is not acting lightheartedly, cruelly, or disrespectfully, but has already learned, or is learning, how to behave as a physician. He is developing in himself the objectivity and the feelings of detached concern that are so necessary to effective clinical work. The student, however, is just beginning to feel and know the deep anxieties, the fears, and the anguish of the physician. He is becoming dimly aware that disintegration and death await both patient and healer, and that physicians are only men, not supermen. The distortions in his perception of the behavior of house staff and physicians are understandable. To explain and correct such distortions, however, requires teachers who can perceive and differentiate the appropriate or inappropriate behavior of their colleagues. (This inaccurate view of the medical staff was not present in residents and practitioners.)

3. It was important, too, for the instructors to understand the difficult role of the resident on a busy medical and surgical ward. It appeared that the psychiatric teacher tended to have a distorted view of the functioning of the medical house staff, especially since he was so far removed from the resident's world of responsibility. It became clear that, like the students, the instructors too had fears and anxieties about the dying patient and the incurable patient.

As these issues became more apparent and were dealt with by open discussion, it seemed to the supervisor that it would be most appropriate and important to include medical residents as instructors for the students. One reason for including medical residents was to give the instructors as well as the supervisor a better idea of what actually went on in the medical wards and emergency room; but the most important reason was to introduce a new method of teaching for the medical

[239]

resident by changing his role from a passive one (as student) to an active one (as teacher). Currently, one of the medical residents, who was a resident-student in the program during the previous year, has joined the group as a teacher and has already contributed a great deal to the supervisory sessions.

THE INTRODUCTION OF THE INSTRUMENT: THE PRECIPITATING FACTOR OUTLINE

About a year ago the group responsible for the family-physician teaching program (Drs. Milton Rosenbaum, Wil Tanenbaum, and David Mann) attempted to devise some method of evaluating the program. During the deliberations the senior author arbitrarily decided that the most important task facing the group was not to evaluate the program, since we were convinced that it had been effective, but rather to introduce techniques and methods into the armamentarium of the physician that he could use as an "instrument." Actually in 1961 a structured interview designed to evaluate the family physicians' seminars had been given to the family physicians and a small group of third-year medical students and first-year medical residents who had participated in the teaching sessions previously described. One item asked the respondents to estimate the effect of the conferences on their knowledge of "total medicine." It was most striking to find that, while everyone answered the question easily, all of the residents and medical students and about half of the physicians spontaneously took exception to the wording of the question. The sense of their reaction seemed to be that, while useful, the material in the course should not be called "knowledge." Perhaps this particular response may point to a more general view of psychosocial material—it is interesting, and sometimes useful, but is rather alien to their field of operation. Such responses strengthened our desire to find an "instrument" which could be incorporated into the physician's existing frame of reference.

The "instrument," which obviously had to be concerned with history-taking and interviewing, was developed in the following way: the senior author, an experienced and "effective" interviewer, knew that there was nothing magical in his method and that the information he attempted to get was available to anyone. He jotted down on a piece of paper those areas that he explored during an interview. He then held a meeting with the family physicians, in which he told them that, since they had been observing him interview patients for several years, he wondered what in their opinion, were the most important topics to be sought out in trying to assess the role of emotional and psychological factors in a patient's illness. In an hour's discussion, the family physicians brought out each and every point that he himself had considered relevant. Thus a simple device was created for the purpose of encouraging them to use this information in their contacts with patients. The "instrument" (Table 1) was worked out with the advice of the entire seminar group. In all, three seminars were devoted to as thorough a discussion as possible of all the considerations which might complicate the family doctor's efforts to apply these simple but sound psychological principles in his medical practice. The main problem, as usual, was that sufficient time was not available for an adequate exploration of the patient's feelings, even though it was emphasized that in the majority of cases the use of the "instrument" would require less than five minutes. We were quite aware of the importance of the "time factor" to the physician. Certainly, "the lack of time" or "the length of

[241]

time necessary for psychological exploration" can become an excuse for resistance; but the teacher must respect the reality of this frequent complaint. Therefore, right from the start, we structured all interviews and examinations of patients so as to be within the time limit that the physicians allowed for patients, about one-half hour for new patients, and 10 to 15 minutes for return visits.

TABLE 1

THE PRECIPITATING FACTOR FORM

1) The precipitating factor of the present illness (the main question is to determine why the patient got sick or suffered a relapse or exacerbation at *this particular time*)

   (a) Any recent losses or separations (deaths, births, children leaving, moves, sickness in others who are meaningful to patient, etc.)
     YES _____ NO _____

   If yes, describe:

2) How are things going at home? (Write the verbatim answer)

3)   *MOTHER*   *FATHER*
   Living _____ Dead _____   Living _____ Dead _____

   (a) If living:
      Sick _____ Well _____   Sick _____ Well _____

      If sick:
      Diagnosis _____   Diagnosis _____

   (b) If dead:
      Date _____ Age _____   Date _____ Age _____
      Type of illness

   Age of *patient* when parent died: _____

4) Anniversary reactions: YES _____ NO _____
   If yes, describe:

5) Identification in choice of symptoms: YES _____ NO _____
   If yes, describe:

6) In your opinion, are emotional factors associated with the illness at this time?
       YES _____ NO _____
   Comments:

[242]

The concern about time also appears to be a reflection of the doctor's lack of confidence in his ability to terminate an interview with comfort. Evidence for this interpretation is contained in one doctor's report on a precipitating factors form: "This patient has pertinent features, but let me tell you, I'm seeing her one hour and twenty minutes beyond her scheduled appointment. I was supposed to be finished with all my patients half an hour ago. I still have four more patients to see—I can't be a working machine and do this sort of work." The medical students also felt such a psychological investigation, no matter how brief, was a threat to the crucially important matter of taking the medical history, as they feared that the patient, like the "crocks" that plagued their lives, might go on talking endlessly about trivial social and family matters, while they were under pressure of time to get a pertinent medical history to present to their teachers. Like the family doctors, they were afraid that once turned on, a patient could not be turned off.[1]

The family doctors were requested to use the precipitating-factors form for a period of approximately two months. The results of this trial run revealed that in a group of 174 patients, the majority of them seen for routine physical examination, about one-half were without noticeable emotional problems (items 1 and 2 in the precipitating factors form). In the other half, an equal number of patients were found with nonspecific problems, on the one hand, and identification or anniversary reactions on the other.

Now for a few words about the "instrument." We have compared it with other instruments which physicians use regularly, such as the stethoscope. We believe that there is

[1] Psychiatrists handle this by the structured "fifty"-minute hour.

[243]

a natural inclination in the physician to look for pathology. A good doctor is always looking for the abnormal. Though he may find a lesion but rarely, he always performs his physical examination, and he uses his stethoscope to keep an ear out for signs of trouble. And what is his reaction when he does uncover a pathological sign, say, an abnormal heart murmur, a Babinski, or a choked disc? The initial feeling is one of gratification and even excitement, as if a discovery were made. The important point here is to keep in mind the physician's strong need of finding something—that is, psysicians are primarily interested in disease. By using our "instrument," the doctor has a tool with which he can examine the critical areas of his patient's psychological life, just as with his stethoscope, he can examine vital organs; and, by having an effective instrument which he can learn to master, he increases his chances of uncovering relevant material and thus satisfying his need to detect concealed pathology.

In our teaching we emphasize that the physician who utilizes such a psychological instrument must be prepared to identify and control the feelings aroused in him by the material he elicits. It is not reasonable to expect a medical student or a practitioner to deal as objectively with a finding, say, of parental rejection, as he would with the discovery of a heart murmur; and he must be taught to recognize the importance of his own feelings in determining the manner in which a psychological finding is to be handled. We know, however, that psychological factors in illness are often left unexplored because of a physician's unconscious need to avoid arousing disturbing feelings in himself. By utilizing the "instrument," the doctor can employ a routine and objective technique to help him overcome his own emotional resistances, and thus proceed with an investigation that otherwise might not have been undertaken.

A related issue concerns the psychiatrist's attitude to himself as a citizen and to the place of psychological data in medical practice. Many nonpsychiatric physicians are most conversant and interested in the broad social, cultural, ethical, intellectual and political aspects of life, despite the fact that as medical men they may give the opposite impression. Such people cannot be reached by an attitude implying that they are inferior social beings as compared to the psychiatrist, and that their data are of a lower order of significance—in other words, that they are the "bad guys" and we are the "good guys." Rather, it seems to us that in order to be effective as teachers of psychological medicine we must relate to them as colleagues who, by sharing our knowledge and understanding of human psychology, can increase their functional capacity as physicians. When we discuss the role of psychological factors in medicine, or the use of our "instrument," the emphasis should be on the finding and the understanding of pathology and on indications for treatment. If in the process some students grow and develop as human beings, so much the better, but this is not our aim.

One final word. How does one answer the question, "What do I do now?" or "What do I do next?" brought up by the medical resident, the physician, and also the student after he develops some understanding of what we are about, or, in other words, after he uses the "instrument" and hits pay dirt? I have answered by using the medical model and by asking another question: "What would you do if through your stethoscope you heard some unusual heart sound? You might ask for further tests; you might ask the patient to return within a week for re-examination; you might immediately request a consultation with a cardiologist; or you might decide to follow the patient in the hope that you will gain further understanding of the meaning of the physical finding and therefore be in a better position to institute the most adequate therapeutic program." And so it is, we believe, with the use of the "psychological instrument,"[2] with one essential difference: once the physician has learned something about the precipitating factors of the illness as well as the general psychological and emotional status of the patient, then he is not only in a position to increase his understanding of the problem, but the very process of obtaining the information may be therapeutic in itself. The personal satisfaction that the physician feels in "finding something," which in turn allows for potential mastery of a problem which might have caused him to feel helpless and even hopeless, then can become a powerful force in strengthening or improving the doctor-patient relationship and in stimulating him to include a more active psychological approach in the total therapeutic program.

[2] Obviously our "instrument," unlike the stethoscope, is discarded after "it" becomes incorporated into the physician's armamentarium in an automatic manner. This is similar to the "brief neurological screening examination," which can be done by a well-trained physician without resort to the "neurological examination form" of his student and resident days.

Discussion

DR. VALENSTEIN: The title of this Symposium was originally phrased as the question, "Can psychiatry be taught?" I feel sure that no reply in the unqualified negative or positive was expected. More likely, the question was intended to elicit the specificities with regard to the teaching of dynamic psychiatry, when and to what extent, to whom and under what circumstances it is best taught. Implicit in our reappraisal of the teaching of dynamic psychiatry is the possibility of isolating the elements that favor or hinder such teaching. If we arrive at some answers, we will have done enough, even though we may have to ask the question again in 30 years.

PROFESSOR ERIKSON: When it comes to medical house officers and doctors in private practice, I know them only as analysands, or indeed as one of their medical patients, that is, the kind of creature who according to Dr. Zinberg was just wheeled into surgery and turns out to be "an excellent example" of one thing or another, and who gives Dr. Rosenbaum's doctor that exquisite personal satisfaction of "finding pathology." While it would be good to have some patients as well as some house

Professor Erik H. Erikson, Drs. Henry Fox, and Paul G. Meyerson delivered prepared discussions by invitation.

Drs. Milton Rosenbaum, Albert J. Solnit, John P. Spiegel, and Helene Deutsch took part in the general discussion.

officers represented in a symposium like this one, it does not seem to be my mandate to speak for the patient. If I then ask myself why I was invited to discuss these papers, I think it was because we are being asked to consider morality, values, and identity; thus I will try to say something about morality and identity.

Let me be a little challenging. When Dr. Zinberg speaks of Freud's "indifference to ethics," his remarks may well be misunderstood. We know what he means. But we also know that, in the popularization of psychoanalysis, this misunderstanding has played a major role, and has in fact led to a misuse of psychoanalytic insight as a justification of immoral or amoral behavior. Freud was in fact an extremely moral man, so much so, that he could say, "I take morality for granted." He took it so much for granted that he would not take—or approve of our taking—any patient for psychoanalytic treatment whom he did not consider a relatively moral person. Freud was tolerant of people with strong conflicts; he was not tolerant of moral weaklings.

In following Freud's precepts, I think we do not tolerate immorality, except as a *symptom of conflict in a moral person*. On the other hand, Dr. Zinberg was quite right in saying that Freud was a severe critic of such moralities or moralisms as make it really impossible for any decent and intelligent person to be both moral and healthy. What is more, he provided the evidence and the theory on the basis of which the autocracy of moral systems can be questioned.

This much about a possible misunderstanding. I know, of course, that Dr. Zinberg meant to discuss psychotherapeutic procedure and not philosophy. I wonder how many of the values he proposed are really methodological necessities. For example, if we pay attention to the whole life cycle of a person when we try to judge a personality symptom, that is really a methodological necessity for us. So is our restraint in moral condemnation when we investigate (by the method of free association) the conflicts, the ambivalences, and ambiguities of a patient. If we ask what values underlie such new methodological necessities, I would say that I recognize a combination of open-minded attention, honesty, and respect for the individual ego.

The important factor, then (mentioned by both speakers), is the relationship of such underlying values to the need of each trainee both for competency in method and for identity of personal style. And if the trainee wants to be honest, systematic, *and* helpful in his diagnostic capacity and in his choice of treatment methods, he will have to know something about the method and the findings of psychoanalysis. For if we want to make (as Dr. Zinberg puts it) "ambivalence available for insight," then we have to establish very definite conditions under which ambivalence cannot find a new hiding place.

Yet whenever we try to teach something about these values to students, for whom such values have not yet become part of a professional identity—and this concerns undergraduates as well as medical students—we come up against a resistance which has not been fully dealt with in this conference. This basic resistance is often hidden behind the specific resistances against insight into sexual or aggressive wishes or thoughts. In fact, many people today accept such wishes or thoughts far too easily, while retaining the basic resistance to which I am referring. This is the recognition that, in vital matters of decision, we are not functioning according to the dictates of "free will" or according to the logic of the secondary process. The first shock in any confrontation with psychoanalytic

[249]

thought concerns not its content, but the fact that there is *that* much we do *not* know about ourselves. Furthermore, whenever we speak about psychoanalytic method, we (both teachers and students) are always emotionally involved; and it is important to realize that what we call transference and countertransference in therapy is also an inescapable part of teaching, not only as between teacher and student, but also as between teacher and teacher, and student and student. The fact that this is not systematically acknowledged often causes that ambivalent and ambiguous atmosphere which expresses itself in strange tensions, not to speak of gossip and professional antagonisms. What helps here is the continued joy of work itself, the original detection of connections between relevant phenomena which no other science has ever linked more relevantly. What does not help is the dogmatic reiteration that ours is a science among other sciences. For the shock I was speaking about cannot and should not be avoided, and can only be creatively absorbed. In the light of all this, I would paraphrase Dr. Bibring's quotation, "Elementary, Watson," to read, "Elemental, Watson, elemental!"

Now to come to the question of identity: you are probably as tired of this word as I am. It has already become what some people call an "ashcan concept," hospitable to all manner of trash, as well as to some valuable insights which should not be thrown away so carelessly. In particular, one aspect of identity—the negative identity—needs to be considered much more carefully. Dr. Zinberg pointed out that analysts, too, conceive of themselves as "different" when they teach in medical school. I could well imagine that this may have to do with a double-take: "Who, me, going against the tradition of free will and logical determinism?" No wonder, for they once went to medical school themselves and did so in their formative years, when their identity was cast with that admixture of a medical ideology which is the result of one of the strongest and in some ways most monastic of indoctrinations. But then, for them, there followed a second, equally demanding indoctrination, and one which, as I just pointed out, undermined some of the very bases of a scientific and Hippocratic training.

One is always nostalgic for one's earlier identity, even if one must repudiate parts of it constantly or reconvert it to make it a part, the more inclusive identity, of one's later development. I do not mean to single out doctors in this respect (some of my best friends are doctors), and to use myself as an example. I am sure my writings show only too clearly how my earlier role of artist struggles for recombination with my later experience as an analyst. But we are speaking here of medical school, and I wonder whether a certain nostalgia for an earlier, more strictly medical identity may at times make it difficult to avoid identifying with the demands of the students' resistance, by representing the mind too mechanically and too practically, or, on the other hand, to identify with their all too fanatic conversion to psychoanalytic thinking. Students, regardless of their level, must gain from us some kind of shock experience. Dr. Kubie has called it a therapeutic experience, but I am not sure that this is the right expression. It has also been called a maturation experience, but I am not sure about that phrase either, because the experience is really a very specific one. The student should learn to experience the possibility that, in his functioning identity, he may combine traditional medical concerns with a totally new kind of insight, not only one needed for the understanding of certain symptoms, but also one that cannot help revolutionizing one's views of man—including oneself.

[251]

DR. FOX: From his experience in teaching medical house officers, Dr. Zinberg has clearly described certain differences in their approach to a patient as compared to that of the psychiatrist. These observations seem useful and quite valid. His deliberate emphasis on a value system of psychoanalytic psychiatry in conflict with the value system of other professional groups, on the other hand, provokes the kind of discussion he presumably expected.

As Heinz Hartmann (1960) reminded us in his lecture, "Psychoanalysis and Moral Values," Freud did not believe that psychoanalysis is in a position to create a philosophy of life, but he clearly saw that the relation of analysis to value problems was of necessity the same as that of any other science. Hartmann later remarked that it is helpful for the analyst to keep himself aware of the difference between his general moral code and his professional code. In his therapeutic work he will keep other values in abeyance and concentrate on the realization of one category of values only: health values.

Thus psychoanalytic psychiatrists and physicians in other specialties share the fundamental values of science and health. Differences emerge from the ways in which these values are defined and combined. For example, Dr. Maxwell Gitelson has stated that we are caught in an identity conflict between psychiatry, which is a therapeutic specialty of medicine, and psychoanalysis, which is a basic science. Dr. Gitelson has expressed concern that therapeutic investment may submerge scientific development. Other psychoanalysts continue to share the view of most physicians who regard the values of science and health as intimately related. Eissler, for instance, has recently referred to Freud's five case histories as the pillars on which psychoanalysis as an empirical science rests.

[252]

Eissler adds that the deep impression left on the reader by these case histories is, among other things, a result of their being descriptions of something *perceived,* not deduced.

House officers, medical students, and also psychiatric residents all respond enthusiastically to the demonstration of what can be perceived during an interview with a patient. Dr. Rosenbaum has reported the favorable impression on medical residents when the psychiatrist interviewed a young man with ulcerative colitis and brought out fresh, relevant historical information. After the instructor had demonstrated his interviewing technique, the residents did the interviewing themselves in later sessions, and apparently no conflict in value systems interfered with the success of this teaching exercise.

What can be perceived does, of course, depend on the outlook of the perceiver, and the technique of interviewing results to a large extent from assumptions concerning what may be revealed during a conversation with a physician, in which the patient is encouraged to use his own language and associations. In her article on psychiatry and medical practice in the general hospital, Dr. Bibring has described the psychiatrist's viewpoint, which maintains that there is more to a person's emotional processes than appears on the surface, and that his behavior patterns and attitudes are the results of conflicts between his deep strivings and his defensive methods against these strivings, developed in a slow adaptive process under the impact of environmental pressures and demands. Illness, as she points out, has to be understood as a stress situation which threatens the psychologic equilibrium and revives patterns of conflict established during the individual's earlier development.

Dr. Grete L. Bibring's remarks lucidly illustrate the struc-

[253]

tural rather than the topographic concept of human personality, and she emphasizes the conflict between strivings and defenses, whether or not they happen to be conscious or unconscious. Since defense patterns such as denial or intellectualization can easily be observed while one is taking a medical history, the nonpsychiatrist can accept their reality and consider their implications without feeling that his value system as a medical scientist has been challenged. Moreover, when the nonpsychiatrist has been encouraged to record the patient's full verbatim statement of his complaint, he can often convincingly demonstrate the reemergence of fears and fantasies from long ago. This focus on the communication of current thoughts and feelings characterizes a good history by a medical house officer as effectively as a psychoanalytic session, and it certainly involves no clash in values.

The extent to which an understanding of a patient's psychological state and its relationship to all his experiences should be pursued would seem to depend on the practical requirements of the job at hand, rather than on the value system of the physician. Here again, the presenting complaint needs careful evaluation from what might be considered a structural point of view—specifically, to what extent the complaint represents local and to what extent organismic dysfunction involving the response of the person and his individual history.

Dr. Rosenbaum's emphasis on the immediate setting for the present illness and on the minimum facts concerning the members of the family constellation certainly helps the nonpsychiatrist to obtain the information he needs for the diagnosis and treatment of the patient. The effect is to broaden rather than to greatly lengthen the history. This would seem to correspond very well with the values of science and health shared by psychiatrists as well as nonpsychiatrists.

Some nonpsychiatrists feel an urge to be men of action, and psychoanalytically oriented psychiatrists (especially during the early phases of their training) sometimes feel that they should avoid this tendency. The nature of their identification with their teachers and perhaps the characteristics of their personal defenses certainly influence their behavior. But the value system of both psychiatrists and nonpsychiatrists would surely require that the patient be given as much direction as he really needs and no more. This might at times require a diet, a drug, or even enforced hospitalization. The training of the psychoanalytic psychiatrist, one hopes, increases his flexibility without necessarily changing his basic professional values.

Nonpsychiatrists as well as psychiatrists try to avoid allowing their moral judgment to interfere with the professional job of maintaining the patient's health. This may be easier for the psychiatrist because he is acutely aware of the extent to which the patient's moral demands on himself so often interfere with his good health. Furthermore, during his own training the psychoanalytic psychiatrist has presumably had the opportunity of appreciating the complexity of human motivation and of modifying his urge to make moral judgments on the behavior of other people.

House officers in teaching hospitals have a special interest in science and research. They are often chosen because they have special abilities along these lines, and, although they are responsible for the care of patients, many of them feel that this care has secondary importance.

Up to the present time the climate at universities and medical schools has encouraged the consideration of preclinical research as "basic," and clinical research as merely "applied." Observation of the molecular and the microscopic still has the highest and "purest" status. As Dr. Gitelson remarked in his presidential address to the International Psychoanalytic Congress, the prestigious results obtained from the suitable and necessary methods of the physical sciences have made them the criterion of all scientific research. Dr. Gitelson expressed concern that psychoanalysts too have caught the fever, and warned against the tendency for resorting to interdisciplinary research as a remedy for social anxiety.

Dr. Gitelson rightly emphasizes that only within the psychoanalytic situation do psychoanalysts occupy their explicit scientific position for studying their proper material—the unconsciously emerging manifestations of instinct, primary process, affects, conflicts, defense mechanisms, and transferences. But the appropriate investigation of a wide range of problems involving complex psychophysiological relationships requires the collaboration of both psychiatrists and non-psychiatrists.

The advancement of psychoanalysis from topographic to structural concepts has established the necessary background for the participation of psychoanalysts in this kind of project. On the other hand, George Simpson, professor of vertebrate paleontology at Harvard University, has recently reminded us that even physicists have found that at least some of their laws are not invariable; that their predictions are statistical and not precise; that certain observations cannot in fact be made; and that absolute confirmation by testing a hypothesis therefore cannot be obtained. The recognition of the essential complexity of the biological sciences gives those house officers who are headed for careers in research the basis for their helping to design collaborative studies of this type.

DR. VALENSTEIN: Dr. Fox, as I understand it, has reminded us to give the picture a balance, to take note of the values that physicians hold in common, including the physician-trained psychoanalyst and the physician-trained internist or other specialist. He emphasizes this mutuality because it contributes to the formation of a collaborative atmosphere, without which teaching would not be possible. Professor Erikson touched on this subject when he pointed out that included in our final identity as psychoanalysts who teach students or house officers, is our own previous experience of having also been trained as physicians.

DR. MEYERSON: Dr. Zinberg and Dr. Rosenbaum and his colleagues have written very interesting papers, which from different points of view bear on the problems of communication between the psychiatrist and his medical colleagues. Dr. Zinberg's major interest lies in the differing value systems of the two groups: he indicates that the psychiatrist's lack of awareness of this difference leads to a breakdown in communication. Dr. Rosenbaum issues a special caveat lest psychiatrists consider the physician's approach to patients a lower order of significance. He implies that a condescending attitude will lead to an alienation of the physicians whom the psychiatrist is trying to help. His own "psychological instrument" should, he suggests, be utilized as a means for structuring the confusion that the physician otherwise experiences when he attempts to understand the nature of his patient's psychological problems. He does not believe that the psychiatrist's primary aim in teaching medical residents is fostering their growth and development as human beings for he apparently feels that this goal implies a lack of respect for their potentialities and talents.

Both papers make significant observations which are extremely relevant to the difficulties frequently encountered in teaching medical residents. In any discussion about the difficulties in communication between the psychiatrist and his colleagues, we are confronted with the discomforting fact that the major obstacles to the physician's increased understanding of psychological problems are his own anxiety and resentment stirred up by his patient's behavior. To use Dr. Zinberg's examples, a physician finds it hard to understand why a juvenile diabetic patient refuses to take his insulin, for the most part because such behavior makes him angry and anxious. No amount of encouragement to discuss the emotional impact of an organic illness will avail if the physician, as is so often the case, feels helpless and frustrated when he cannot find tangible means to cure his patients medically. It is perfectly true, as both presentors indicate, that the physician's anxiety is compounded when we urge him to play a role that is often poorly defined and when we expect him to use concepts that are sometimes nebulous even to psychiatrists who have invested considerable amounts of energy trying to understand them. We ourselves—the psychiatrists—have marked difficulty in feeling comfortable in many of the stressful relationships we encourage our students to set up with emotionally disturbed medical patients. Yet, above and beyond the urgency of the physician's reality, the demands of his training, his necessarily circumscribed interest, and his differing value system, it is his own attitudes which are mobilized by contact with patients who are upset that play the dominant part in his difficulty in absorbing psychological concepts.

[258]

Can we, therefore, be effective in teaching medical residents, if we do not try in some way to modify those attitudes that disturb the relationships they have with their patients? What understanding can the physician really assimilate and utilize if he continues to be frightened and angry? In an ad hoc situation in which we as psychiatrists are called in consultation for a particular crisis, we are naturally patient-oriented. We suggest measures that we hope will alleviate the patient's suffering and we take into consideration the realities that confront the patient and his physician. However, when we have an opportunity to teach psychological concepts to young interns or residents, our aims usually are quite different. We become physician-oriented, and in one way or another try to modify those attitudes and behaviors of our student-colleagues that we believe interfere with their practice of medicine. Our basic problem in this type of teaching is to create a climate in which our goal of modulating the physician's unfruitful attitudes can be achieved. Inevitably, any discussion of patient's psychological conflicts, no matter how didactic and structured, mobilizes emotional responses in the physician and threatens his understanding of what we are attempting to illustrate. Drs. Wermer and Stock have discussed this issue in their paper and have delineated their attempts to foster a constructive psychiatrist-pediatrician relationship, which they feel is crucial for mastering the psychological concepts they proffer to the pediatrician. Action or attitudes on the part of the psychiatrist that either seriously antagonize his students and medical colleagues, or markedly intensify their anxiety, clearly do not promote the appropriate climate for a modification of unhealthy attitudes toward patients.

I wonder if part of our difficulty in stating this issue more directly stems from our concern as to whether we have the right to modify someone else's attitudes, especially if that someone is not asking to have his attitudes changed. Dr. Zinberg has warned quite rightly against the danger of a psychiatrist merchandising truth at all costs. To paraphrase what he says: the psychiatrist who zealously attempts to impose upon others his own belief that extensive self-knowledge is universally good becomes a zealot, and a zealot is a better propagandist than a teacher. Behavior of this type is not based upon a relative system of beliefs—Dr. Zinberg's definition of values. In addition to its being bad manners, it does not achieve its goal. A psychiatrist usually behaves dogmatically with physicians for the same reason that physicians act this way with their patients, i.e., he is anxious and he anticipates their resentment, whether it is forthcoming or not.

Dr. Zinberg discusses this issue in terms of conflicting values. His approach is very stimulating and makes a needed point, which is driven home (often inexorably and painfully) in most experienced psychiatric teachers. Nonetheless, it is possible for a psychiatrist to present a new point of view about patient care and even to indicate his own value system as related to various medical situations, without imposing these values upon his students. Attitudes about patients are on the open market; the medical student, the house officer, and the medical resident are constantly exposed by their teachers to a variety of responses to patients. Medical personnel are perfectly free to choose the approach that suits them best, and the psychiatrist, I believe, is free to compete for their attention. The psychiatrist who teaches obviously feels it is of value to teach, and I do not think we can get away from the fact that explicitly or implicitly he feels it is valuable for a physician to have less anxious and less angry attitudes toward his patients.

If you will permit me to be dogmatic, I would like to affirm my belief that it is both necessary and legitimate to attempt to modify medical residents' attitudes. There are various techniques for accomplishing this goal, granting that we can be successful in this effort only to a limited extent with any resident, and partially successful with only a limited number of residents. It is not so much what one does but the way one does it. Because of a variety of tactical problems relevant to the local scene—the New England Center Hospital—I have found it of great help to interview personally a considerable number of patients, over a period of time, in the presence of the residents. I obviously try in this way to present myself as a nonthreatening model for identification. I certainly make every effort at all times to show respect and tolerance for the patients I interview and to avoid as much as possible becoming anxious and angry. However, on what I consider appropriate occasions, I indicate the universality of anxious and angry responses and suggest various ways of managing these reactions in oneself. Of course, an understanding of what is bothering the patient, especially if he brings out this information during the interview, helps both the residents and myself feel less threatened. It is, however, my impression that this understanding is secondary to the effect I achieve through revealing my own attitudes toward the patients I interview. I try to say in a low-pitched manner: "This is the way I do it; I am showing you a possible approach to the understanding and possible management of patients which you might consider; I hope you do." In any case, I try to maintain my role as *a teacher who respects his students yet recognizes that they have a lot to learn.*

I think it is clear that I am drawing on analogies with psychotherapeutic techniques as a basis for modifying the resi-

[261]

dents' attitudes toward their patients. I am not suggesting that psychiatrists conduct group therapy with medical residents. I would like to reemphasize, however, the value of developing a relationship between teacher and student in which there is mutual respect. I think also that if the psychiatrist can communicate his appreciation of the difficulties which the resident does experience when he is confronted with the emotional disturbances of his patients, particularly as the psychiatrist reveals some aspects of his own difficulties, he will make his message more meaningful and more palatable.

If we scratch deeply enough in situations in which a recalcitrant patient makes his physician angry, we will find that the roots of this reaction reside in the latter's frustrated narcissism or disappointed rescue fantasies. If these roots are powerful enough, nothing the psychiatrist does as a teacher will diminish the rage and anxiety that the resident or the physician feels. However, if changes in attitudes can occur without the interpretation and working through of unconscious conflicts—which I believe is possible with many people —the approach I have described may aid some physicians to a better toleration of their own and their patients' anger and anxiety. Clearly, a knowledge as to why a patient is angry or upset, and the availability of techniques such as the one Dr. Rosenbaum uses which help structure otherwise chaotic psychological material, are most helpful in diminishing that component of the resident's anxiety which stems from lack of understanding. It may well be that for certain types of residents, as Dr. Rosenbaum implies, didactic methods suffice, and once the resident's uncertainty about what he is doing is alleviated, he will reorient his attitudes toward his patients in the natural process of maturation without needing the psychiatrist as a model for identification. Part of the psychiatrist's problem in teaching residents parallels the resident's difficulty with his patients: he is in a very open-ended, unscientific situation, without adequate controls or even adequate follow-up studies. If he is going to function at all in a new situation, he must draw upon his own experiences with people in a variety of relationships and use those methods that suit him and make sense to him. I find I function most successfully when I employ the measures I have described.

DR. VALENSTEIN: Dr. Myerson has not only introduced a welcome note of optimism at this final point of our Symposium, but he has also clarified matters by recalling that, although teachers carry common values in their approach, each arranges them according to his own individual temperament and perspective. Respect for the individuality of the student and of the teacher is a paramount value, just as it is in therapeutic relationships, between the doctor and his patient.

* * *

DR. ROSENBAUM: I agree with Professor Erikson when he speaks about the methodological necessities of doctors and psychiatrists as opposed to values. If I emphasize self-knowledge to the medical students and to the house officers, I emphasize this not because it is particularly valuable. Actually, this is the necessary condition for the practice of medicine, that is all. If you want to be a baker or a banker, you do not even have to try to remember a fantasy. It makes no difference to your clients. But if you are going to be a doctor, it might. As a doctor, I do not care whether you beat your wife or whether you are a Republican. Next week, however, I am going to do in New York what I used to do in Cincinnati: before the elections, I would make rounds and ask every patient on the wards whether he was a Republican or a Democrat; if he turned out to be a Republican, I would say that we had better keep him in.

In Cincinnati, we used to have a group psychosomatic conference consisting of eight or nine students; it was a sort of bull session. I recall an occasion when eight senior students were in my office and one of them asked how to go about getting an autopsy. So I said, "Okay, how *do* you get an autopsy?" Then, to my surprise, three of the eight students said they would not let anybody in their families undergo an autopsy. They had seen what took place at the Cincinnati General Hospital; how bodies were strewn about and butchered up. How should I have handled this situation? I could have said, "You know, this attitude simply means you're a sadist. You wanted to kill your brother, sister, father, and mother. That's why you are against an autopsy." I did not say that. Instead, I said, "You know, I'm very proud and happy that you've been so honest. But you have to remember that next year you're going to be an intern, and you're going to be expected to get autopsies. Now, if you cannot keep your own feelings out of it, I can assure you that you are not going to get an autopsy, because you are going to communicate this to the family. This is why many interns do not get autopsies. So what can you do? You can do only one of two things. You can somehow master this yourself. You do not have to go into analysis. But the fact that you are aware of these feelings and will give them a little thought may help you. If not, do not try to get an autopsy. Tell your resident to get the autopsy, because you are not going to get it. It is that simple."

I think I learned a great deal from Professor Erikson's fine remarks, especially in regard to the nostalgia for our old identities. Perhaps this nostalgia explains my fantasy of what I want to do on my sabbatical—be an intern in the emergency room. It is interesting to note that whenever psychoanalysts get together at a conference on how to train psychiatric residents, we emphasize that we do not teach residents enough clinical psychiatry. Why do we emphasize this? Because this is what the residents yearn for. Why did we go into medicine? The reasons that made us go into medicine have nothing to do with understanding people. They have to do with mastering anxieties on the deepest levels, through action. It is our effort to beat the game of life, our effort to prevent our own death. That's why we go into medicine. Then we have to master something else: passivity versus activity.

DR. SOLNIT: After hearing Dr. Rosenbaum, I remembered Dr. Kaufman's description of the need to teach certain things over and over again. He said it was like pushing a heavy boulder up an inclined plane, making only a few inches of progress at a time, then losing a few inches when he got tired. There is another way of looking at it. There are certain kinds of plants that have to be planted each year, nourished each year, and enjoyed each year. Other plants do not have to be pampered, but must be nourished and helped to grow larger and stronger by being provided with the proper kind of environment. So, if you are feeling pessimistic, you can say that the questions asked 30 years ago are still pertinent today— perhaps the only difference is that today they are being asked more specifically and more fruitfully. I hope we can pass on to the next generation the same questions, with modifications, so that they will be increasingly useful as questions.

Although Dr. Kaufman reminded us that we should not forget the past, I think that we should also keep in mind that we have the responsibility and the opportunity to benefit

[265]

from the past in order to enrich the present as well as the future. So the same questions may have to be answered as well as reformulated every year. Sometimes at the end of a long day or at the end of a long year I would like to say, "Now that question is answered and I am finished." The truth is that we cannot be finished because certain kinds of human conditions cannot be wrapped up and put away. I myself am very grateful that they cannot be. Also, I would like to remind you that we have to recruit people into our field. Not everyone is eager to come into it, until they know more of what we represent. That is why models are most important—the human models, the Dr. Bibrings, the Professor Eriksons, the Dr. Loewensteins. Out of these come other kinds of questions and approaches which we can use to exploit the continuity of past and present. The naturalist model is a demanding and fruitful one; the pattern of applying theory to refine the theory, and to uncover and translate new knowledge is vitally important. We are not yet very skillful at translating, and to explain this as a resistance is inaccurate and fruitless. If we asked our pediatric friends and colleagues, they could just as easily accuse us of being resistant to knowing what the realities of pediatric practice are. I would like to take particular exception to the idea that these applications of theory are based mainly on ideologies. The crucial considerations should deal with the scientific characteristics of our data and how they are applied.

DR. SPIEGEL: I am grateful to Dr. Myerson and to Dr. Zinberg for demonstrating two major but contradictory positions which can be taken with respect to values. The difference lies between those who take a relative and those who take an absolute view of values. In spite of several qualifications, Dr. Myerson seemed to be speaking for the absolute view whereas Dr. Zinberg was trying to illustrate the advantage of the relative view in which values are seen to vary quite legitimately in accordance with the social and cultural characteristics of defined groups. Dr. Zinberg was saying, in effect, "One set of values governs the patterning of the professional roles of medical personnel, another set legitimizes the roles of psychiatrists. Neither is right or wrong, and both may work well enough in their separate contexts. The discrepancy between them, however, may, and often does, lead to difficulties in communication about and collaboration in the care of patients. The more we are aware of the relativity of the discrepant values, the better we can cope with the resultant problems." Dr. Myerson, on the other hand, seemed to be saying, "My values are correct; I am hopeful that they will prevail, and I will act upon them to the best of my ability in my relations with other medical specialties, because I look at their values as something to be changed for the better—namely, my values."

The choice between these two positions is an open one and much that has been said in the course of this conference reflects one or the other choice. As for myself, I would agree with Dr. Zinberg that the relative position and the attempt to be precise about value differences reduces conflict between the professions and makes communication problems easier to handle. It removes the tone of authority and superiority often responsible for "resistance" to psychiatrists.

On the score of "resistance," I would like to second Dr. Solnit's suggestion that we resist using "resistance" as a catch-all word for explaining all our problems in communication. This practice overloads the word to such a degree as to rob it of all its technical meaning. It does not make sense for a Re-

[267]

publican to say, in the course of a political campaign, that the Democrats are resisting him—or that they have an unconscious need to be Democrats—when the two parties are chiefly proceeding from different value assumptions and ideologies. The word is important enough to preserve it for those unconscious conflicts that we are working out with patients. If, in our relations with other professionals, we could disregard their emotional conflicts and concentrate on the cognitive and value problems to be worked out with them, our communications would be much more successful.

DR. DEUTSCH: While sitting in the audience, I felt myself to be in a unique position. I had the full objectivity of the audience, while at the same time I had the full identification with my colleagues who undertook this work. There is a certain period in life when a person is apt to be more historically minded, that is, when one has a short future and a long past. Looking to the future, I share fully Dr. Myerson's optimism because I, more than any of you, am deeply aware of how much has been done in a relatively short time, i.e., in 40 years. When one looks back on the history of psychoanalysis, especially as regards the relationship of psychoanalysis to medicine, one can understand the optimistic feeling of immense achievement.

You have let me participate today in the progress of your work. I want to let you participate in my personal historical experience of 40 years ago. Sometime between 1920 and 1922 (I cannot give an exact date) there was a meeting of the Viennese Medical Society. This was the Supreme Court of medicine, whose judgment constituted the decisive evaluation of scientific work in medicine. My husband, Felix

Deutsch, dared to present a paper on psychosomatic medicine at this meeting. I do not remember the content of the paper. (It is interesting and paradoxical that certain events are remembered much more for their traumatic than for their rational elements.) This was the first lecture in Vienna on psychosomatic medicine and on the relationship of psychoanalysis to medical science. I was sitting with other doctors in the audience. After the lecture, there was a silence so loud that I will never in all my life forget the noise of that silence. I had the feeling that this event was Felix Deutsch's professional death.

Those of you who come from Europe—in this case from Vienna—will more readily understand what kind of politics were involved in an academic career 40 years ago. The big step in such a career was to become *Dozent*. This meant either that one had not been born a Jew, or that he had changed his religion, thereby denying the burdensome past. But even then one's scientific achievement had to be outstanding and recognized.

Felix Deutsch was one of the very few, perhaps the first, whose merits had been accepted without his having to change his religion; but the reaction to his paper, the silence, meant that his academic career was finished. With his escort Felix went to another part of the building, while I walked out of the assembly room with most of the long-bearded professors. Since I was not known in this circle then, they spoke freely about my husband and what he had done. (Although I don't know their names, I remember their faces well.) At first one said, "Why do they let a crazy man speak in this group?" Another replied, "But he has done excellent work in internal medicine!" The man proceeded to comment upon the papers Felix Deutsch had written. After much discussion, they decided, in a spirit of benevolent tolerance, that something had happened to him mentally.

I would like to be able to tell you that I fully appreciated my husband's great courage and that I did not doubt for a moment that he was right. However, I am not quite sure that I can, because at that time my sense of values was not quite stabilized, and I had aspirations for my husband's academic career. I was crushed. At this point the defeated one appeared. He was elated and asked me what I thought about it all. In our talk which followed that Vienna meeting, Felix predicted exactly what we are witnessing here today. When I tell you this story, I do so partly for sentimental reasons, but above all to express my feeling of gratification as to these meetings. They have been born from the combined efforts of your group, and one has the impression that it is only a beginning of the work. From the point of view of the situation 40 years ago, an immense achievement has been made, and I congratulate you!

Bibliography

Alexander, F. and French, T. M. (1946), *Psychoanalytic Therapy*. New York: The Ronald Press.

American Psychiatric Association (1952), *Psychiatry and Medical Education*, Vol. I; *The Psychiatrist: His Training and Development*, Vol. II. Report of the Conferences on Psychiatric Education at Ithaca, New York, 1951 and 1952. Washington: American Psychiatric Association.

American Psychiatric Association, Committee on Medical Education (1956), An Outline for a Curriculum for Teaching Psychiatry in Medical Schools. *Med. Education, 31*: 115.

Becker, H. S., Geer, B., Hughes, E. C., and Strauss, A. M. L. (1961), *Boys in White. Student Culture in Medical School*. Chicago: University of Chicago Press.

Bell, D. (1960), *The End of Ideology*. Glencoe, Ill.: The Free Press.

Benjamin, J. D. (1947), Psychoanalysis and Nonanalytic Psychotherapy. *Psychoanal. Quart., 16*:169-176.

Berman, L. (1949), Countertransferences and Attitudes of the Analyst in the Therapeutic Process. *Psychiat., 12*:159-166.

[271]

Berry, G. P. (1958), Medical Education in Transition. *J. Med. Educat.*, *33*:483-489.

Bibring, E. (1937), Symposium on the Therapeutic Results of Psychoanalysis, VI. *Internat. J. Psycho-Anal.*, *18*:170-189.

—— (1952), Lecture given in a course on ego psychology at the Boston Psychoanalytic Institute.

—— (1954), Psychoanalysis and the Dynamic Psychotherapies. *J. Amer. Psychoanal. Assoc.*, *2*:745-770.

Bibring, G. L. (1947), Psychiatry and Social Work. *J. Soc. Casework, 28*:203-211.

—— (1959), Some Considerations of the Psychological Processes in Pregnancy. In: *The Psychoanalytic Study of the Child, 14*:113-121. New York: International Universities Press.

——, Dwyer, T. F., Huntington, D. S., and Valenstein, A. F. (1961), A Study of the Psychological Processes in Pregnancy and of the Earliest Mother-Child Relationship. *The Psychoanalytic Study of the Child, 16*:9-72. New York: International Universities Press.

Bruner, J. S. (1963), *The Process of Education.* New York: Alfred A. Knopf and Random House, Vintage Books.

Campbell, M. (1930), Psychiatry and the Medical Student. *Psychiat. Quart., 4*:118-132.

Chapman, C. B. (1956), On the Teaching of the Science of Medicine. *Clin. Res. Proceed., 4*:161.

Davidson, H. A. (1964), The Image of the Psychiatrist. *Amer. J. Psychiat., 121*:329.

Deutsch, F., Kaufman, R., and Blumgart, H. L. (1940), Present Methods of Teaching, *Psychosomat. Med., 2*:213-222.

Deutsch, H. (1944-1945), *Psychology of Women,* 2 vols. New York: Grune & Stratton.

Doyle, A. C. (1930), *The Complete Sherlock Holmes.* (Preface by Christopher Morley.) New York: Doubleday and Company.

Erikson, E. H. (1950), *Childhood and Society.* New York: W. W. Norton.

—— (1958), *Young Man Luther.* New York: W. W. Norton.

—— (1959a), The Nature of Clinical Evidence. *Evidence and Inference,* ed. D. Lerner. (The Hayden Colloquium on Scien-

tific Concept and Method.) New York: The Free Press of
Glencoe, pp. 73-96.
——(1959b), Identity and the Life Cycle. *Psychol. Issues,* Monog.
1. New York: International Universities Press.
Evans, L. J. (1963), The Forces That Shape the Medical School.
*J. Med. Educat., 38:*479-484.
Felix, R. H. (1964), The Image of the Psychiatrist, Past, Present,
and Future. *Amer. J. Psychiat., 121:*318-322.
Feuerzweig, W., Munter, P., Swets, J., and Breen, M. (1964),
Computer-Aided Teaching in Medical Diagnosis. *J. Med.
Educat., 39:*746-754.
Freud, A. (1946), *The Ego and the Mechanisms of Defense.* New
York: International Universities Press.
——(1954), Psychoanalysis and Education. Memorial Lecture, de-
livered May 5, 1954, at the New York Academy of Medicine.
In: *The Psychoanalytic Study of the Child, 9:*9-15. New
York: International Universities Press.
——(1958), Adolescence. In: *The Psychoanalytic Study of the
Child, 13:*255-278. New York: International Universities
Press.
——(April 2, 1959), *The Concept of Normality.* Medical Faculty
Lecture: The University of California at Los Angeles.
Freud, S. (1905), Three Essays on the Theory of Sexuality: I. The
Sexual Aberrations. *Standard Edition, 7:*135-245. London:
Hogarth Press.
——(1911), Psycho-analytic Notes on an Autobiographical Ac-
count of a Case of Paranoia (Dementia Paranoides). *Standard Edition, 12:*9-82. London: Hogarth Press.
—— (1915), Papers on Metapsychology. *Standard Edition, 14:*105-
215. London: Hogarth Press.
——(1919), On The Teaching of Psycho-Analysis in Universities.
*Standard Edition, 17:*169.
——(1924), Neurosis and Psychosis. *Standard Edition, 19:*149-153.
Gill, M. M. (1954), Psychoanalysis and Exploratory Psychotherapy. *J. Amer. Psychoanal. Assoc.,* 2:771-797.
Gregg, A. (1948), Limitations of Psychiatry. *Amer. J. Psychiat.,
104:*513.

[273]

Group for the Advancement of Psychiatry, Committee on Medical Education (1948), *Report on Medical Education*. GAP Report No. 3. New York: GAP.

——(1955), *Trends and Issues in Psychiatric Residency Programs*. GAP Report No. 31. New York: GAP.

——(1958), *Small Group Teaching in Psychiatry for Medical Students*. GAP Report No. 40. New York: GAP.

——(1962), *The Preclinical Teaching of Psychiatry*. GAP Report No. 54. New York: GAP.

Ham, G. (1961), Reintegration of Psychoanalysis into Teaching. *Amer. J. Psychiat., 117*:877.

Hartmann, H. (1927), *Die Grundlagen der Psychoanalyse*. Leipzig: Georg Thieme.

——(1939a), Psychoanalysis and the Concept of Health. *Internat. J. Psycho-Anal., 20*:308-321.

——(1939b), *Ego Psychology and the Problem of Adaptation*. New York: International Universities Press, 1958.

——(1953), Contribution to the Metapsychology of Schizophrenia. In: *Essays on Ego Psychology*. New York: International Universities Press, 1964, pp. 182-206.

——, Kris, E., and Loewenstein, R. M. (1953), The Function of Theory in Psychoanalysis. In: *Drives, Affects, Behavior*, Vol. 1, ed. R. M. Loewenstein, New York: International Universities Press, pp. 13-37.

——(1959), Psychoanalysis as a Scientific Theory. In: *Essays on Ego Psychology*. New York: International Universities Press, 1964, pp. 182-206.

——(1960), *Psychoanalysis and Moral Values*. New York: International Universities Press.

Hume, Portia B. (1964), Community Psychiatry, Social Psychiatry, and Community Mental Health Work: Some Intern-Professional Relationships in Psychiatry and Social Work. *Amer. J. Psychiat., 121*:340.

Jones, E. (1955), *The Life and Work of Sigmund Freud*, Vol. 2. New York: Basic Books.

Kahana, R. J. (1959), Teaching Medical Psychology through Psychiatric Consultation. *J. Med. Educat., 34*:1003-1009.

Kahana, R. J. and Bibring, G. L. (1964), Personality Types in Medical Management. In: *Psychiatry and Medical Practice in a General Hospital,* ed. N. E. Zinberg. New York: International Universities Press, pp. 108-123.

Kluckhohn, C. (1951), Values and Value Orientation in the Theory of Action: An Exploration in Definition and Classification. In: *Towards a General Theory of Action,* eds. T. Parsons and E. Shils. Cambridge: Harvard University Press.

Knight, R. P. (1949), A Critique of the Present Status of the Psychotherapies. *Bull. New York Acad. Med., 25*:100-114.

——(1952), An Evaluation of Psychotherapeutic Techniques. *Bull. Menninger Clinic, 16*:113-124.

Kubie, L. S. (1964), Traditionalism in Psychiatry. *J. Nerv. and Ment. Dis., 139*:6-19.

Levine, M. (1942), *Psychotherapy in Medical Practice.* New York: Macmillan.

Lindemann, E. and Dawes, L. G. (1952), The Use of Psychoanalytic Constructs in Preventive Psychiatry. In: *The Psychoanalytic Study of the Child,* 7:429-448. New York: International Universities Press.

Loeb, R. F. (1963), Reflections on Undergraduate Medical Education. *J. Med. Educat., 38*:658-661.

Loewenstein, R. M. (1965), Observational Data and Theory in Psychoanalysis. *Drives, Affects, Behavior,* Vol. 2, ed. M. Schur. New York: International Universities Press, pp. 38-59.

Macalpine, I. (1950), The Development of Transference. *Psychoanal. Quart., 19*:501-539.

MacLeish, A. (1928), The Hamlet of A. MacLeish. In: *Collected Poems 1917-1952.* Boston: Houghton Mifflin Company, 1952, pp. 199-223.

Meyers, M. (1964), The Image of the Psychiatrist. *Amer. J. Psychiat., 121*:323.

Mosel, J. N. (1964), The Learning Process. *J. Med. Educat., 39*: 485-496.

Parsons, T. (1951), *The Social System.* Glencoe, Ill.: The Free Press.

[275]

Pickering, G. (1963), The Present Scope of Medicine. *J. Med. Educat., 38*:681-687.

Rapaport, D. (1960), The Structure of Psychoanalytic Theory. A Systematic Attempt. *Psychol. Issues,* Monog. 6. New York: International Universities Press.

——, and Gill, M. M. (1959), The Points of View and Assumptions of Metapsychology. *Internat. J. Psycho-Anal., 40*:153-162.

Reichard, J. F. (1964), Introduction: The Development and Operation of a Psychiatric Service. *Psychiatry and Medical Practice in a General Hospital,* ed. N. E. Zinberg. New York: International Universities Press.

Sandler, J. (1962), Research in Psychoanalysis. The Hampstead Index as an Instrument of Psychoanalytic Research. *Internat. J. Psycho-Anal., 43*:287.

Solnit, A. J., and Senn, M. J. E. (1954), Teaching Comprehensive Pediatrics in an Outpatient Clinic. *Pediat., 14*:547.

Spencer, H. (1884), *What Knowledge Is of Most Worth.* New York: J. B. Alden.

Spink, W. W. (1964), The Training of the Physician. Continuing Education—Whose Responsibility? *New Eng. J. Med., 271*: 827.

Stone, L. (1951), Psychoanalysis and Brief Psychotherapy. *Psychoanal. Quart., 20*:215-236.

——(1961), *The Psychoanalytic Situation.* New York: International Universities Press.

Szurek, S. (1957), Teaching and Learning of Psychoanalytic Psychiatry in Medical School. *Psychoanal. Quart., 26*:387.

Tidd, C. W. (1960), The Use of Psycho-analytic Concepts in Medical Education. *Internat. J. Psycho-Anal., 41*:559.

Whitehead, A. N. (1929), *The Aims of Education.* New York: Macmillan, 1951.

Whitehorn, J. C. (1963), Education for Uncertainty. *Perspectives in Biology and Medicine, 7*:118-123. Chicago: University of Chicago Press.

Zetzel, E. R. Unpublished papers and lectures.

Zinberg, N. E. (1963), Psychiatry: A Professional Dilemma. *Daedalus,* pp. 808-823.

——(1964a), Introduction: The Development and Operation of a Psychiatric Service. In: *Psychiatry and Medical Practice in a General Hospital,* ed. N. E. Zinberg. New York: International Universities Press.

——(1964b), Psychiatric Rounds on the Private Medical Service of a General Hospital. In: *Psychiatry and Medical Practice in a General Hospital,* ed. N. E. Zinberg. New York: International Universities Press.

——(1965), Psychoanalysis and the American Scene: A Reappraisal. *Diogenes,* no. 50, pp. 73-111.